AF772777

NEPHROLOGY RESEARCH AND CLINICAL DEVELOPMENTS SERIES

NEPHROLOGY - DIALYSIS - TRANSPLANTATION

Nephrology Research and Clinical Developments Series

Nephrology - Dialysis - Transplantation
Endre Krüger and Kelemen Hahn (Editors)
2009 ISBN: 978-1-60741-736-1

NEPHROLOGY RESEARCH AND CLINICAL DEVELOPMENTS SERIES

NEPHROLOGY - DIALYSIS - TRANSPLANTATION

ENDRE KRÜGER
AND
KELEMEN HAHN
EDITORS

Nova Biomedical Books
New York

Copyright © 2009 by Nova Science Publishers, Inc.

All rights reserved. No part of this book may be reproduced, stored in a retrieval system or transmitted in any form or by any means: electronic, electrostatic, magnetic, tape, mechanical photocopying, recording or otherwise without the written permission of the Publisher.

For permission to use material from this book please contact us:
Telephone 631-231-7269; Fax 631-231-8175
Web Site: http://www.novapublishers.com

NOTICE TO THE READER

The Publisher has taken reasonable care in the preparation of this book, but makes no expressed or implied warranty of any kind and assumes no responsibility for any errors or omissions. No liability is assumed for incidental or consequential damages in connection with or arising out of information contained in this book. The Publisher shall not be liable for any special, consequential, or exemplary damages resulting, in whole or in part, from the readers' use of, or reliance upon, this material.

Independent verification should be sought for any data, advice or recommendations contained in this book. In addition, no responsibility is assumed by the publisher for any injury and/or damage to persons or property arising from any methods, products, instructions, ideas or otherwise contained in this publication.

This publication is designed to provide accurate and authoritative information with regard to the subject matter covered herein. It is sold with the clear understanding that the Publisher is not engaged in rendering legal or any other professional services. If legal or any other expert assistance is required, the services of a competent person should be sought. FROM A DECLARATION OF PARTICIPANTS JOINTLY ADOPTED BY A COMMITTEE OF THE AMERICAN BAR ASSOCIATION AND A COMMITTEE OF PUBLISHERS.

Library of Congress Cataloging-in-Publication Data

Nephrology, dialysis, transplantation / editors, Endre Krüger and Kelemen Hahn.
p. ; cm.
Includes bibliographical references and index.
ISBN 978-1-60741-736-1 (hardcover)
1. Kidneys--Diseases. 2. Hemodialysis. 3. Kidneys--Transplantation. I. Krüger, Endre. II. Hahn, Kelemen.
[DNLM: 1. Kidney Diseases. 2. Kidney Transplantation. 3. Renal Dialysis. WJ 300 N439 2009]
RC902.N434 2009
616.6'1--dc22 2009027485

Published by Nova Science Publishers, Inc. ✢ New York

Contents

Preface

Nephrology deals with the study of the function and diseases of the kidney. Autosomal Dominant Polycystic Kidney Disease (ADPKD) is the cause of renal failure in 5-10% of the patients in dialysis or transplantation. This book discusses the several conditions which are associated with the rate of progression. Peritoneal dialysis (PD), which has been widely used as one of the major renal replacement therapies for end-stage renal disease (ESRD) patients is also explored in this book. Furthermore, the important role of PAI-1 and the value of therapeutic approaches targeting PAI-1 in progressive renal fibrosis is also examined. Because renal interstitial fibrosis occurs in virtually all the progressive renal diseases leading to end-stage renal failure, controlling it would be a reasonable therapeutic strategy. Other chapters in this book include a review of therapeutic plasma exchanges (TPE), the potential mechanisms that may regulate the effect of macrophages upon renal interstitial fibrosis and the pathophysiological implications of inflammation in the pathogenesis of diabetic nephropathy.

Chapter I - Diabetes mellitus and diabetic complications have become a major public health problem. One of the most relevant diabetic complications is diabetic nephropathy, which is nowdays the main cause of end-stage renal failure and the leading cause for entry in renal replacement therapy programs. In addition, diabetic nephropathy is associated with a dramatic increase in cardiovascular risk. In spite of the improvement in our knowledge on different aspects of diabetes mellitus, the intimate mechanisms involved in the development and progression of diabetic renal injury are not yet fully known. There is now growing evidence that activation of innate immunity and the subsequent development of a chronic low grade inflammatory reaction are relevant factors in the pathogenesis of diabetes and its complications. There are diverse inflammatory cells, mediators and pathways involved in this scenario, including monocytes/macrophages, lymphocytes, neutrophils, toll-like receptors, chemoattractant cytokines, cell adhesion molecules, and pro-inflammatory cytokines. These factors play a critical role in the development of microvascular diabetic complications, including diabetic nephropathy. This chapter reviews and discusses the pathophysiological implications of inflammation in the pathogenesis of diabetic nephropathy.

Chapter II - Indexing glomerular filtration rate (GFR) for body surface area (BSA) is often realized without arising any questions. However, physiological basis for such an indexation are very poor. Indeed, indexing GFR for BSA to avoid variation due to differences in body size necessarily implies that GFR is a linear function of BSA and that the intercept of this linear function is zero. Moreover, when GFR is indexed for BSA, the relation indexed GFR-BSA must completely disappear. These physiological prerequisites are not found for BSA indexation. The authors will review the history of this indexation and will underline errors and defaults. Different equations to estimate BSA exist and will be discussed. The choice of "1.73 m^2" will be also criticized. Moreover, indexing GFR for BSA has little impact on GFR results in "normal" body size population. Nevertheless, this indexation will have strong consequences in anorexia and in obese patients. These consequences will be illustrated by our original data. The authors will discuss possible alternatives proposed to substitute for BSA indexation.

Chapter III - Peritoneal dialysis (PD) has been widely used as one of the major renal replacement therapies for end-stage renal disease (ESRD) patients. A new PD fluid is instilled into the peritoneal cavity via peritoneal catheter after the previously instilled fluid has been drained out. Exchange of solutes and water between the body and the peritoneal fluid occurs during PD. PD system has three major components – 1) peritoneal fluid compartment, 2) peritoneal microcirculation and 3) peritoneal membrane. Basic mechanism employed in PD lies in diffusion and convection for removing uremic toxins, and ultrafiltration (UF) for water removal. PD fluid contains a high concentration of glucose, which generates an osmotic gradient between the peritoneal fluid and peritoneal microcirculation, resulting in water movement into the peritoneal cavity. There is a wide inter-individual variation in the speed of solute and water transport through the peritoneal membrane. Peritoneal equilibration test (PET) and other tests for the assessment of the peritoneal solute and water transport have been developed. Fast transporters are likely to dissipate osmotic gradient earlier than slow transporters because they absorb glucose more rapidly through the peritoneal membrane. Suspected factors determining the peritoneal solute transport rate (PSTR) are age, diabetes, comorbidity, peritonitis, chronic inflammation and frequent use of bio-incompatible PD fluid containing high glucose and glucose degradation products (GDP). Interleukin-6 (IL-6), vascular endothelial growth factor (VEGF), nitric oxide(NO), cancer antigen 125 (CA125) and transforming growth factor-β (TGF-β) have been associated with PSTR. The role of the genetic polymorphism of the above molecules is under investigation.

The authors have seen remarkable technical advances in the prevention of peritonitis by allowing less chance of contamination during PD fluid exchange (connectology), along with the development of diagnosis and management protocols. Automated PD facilitating fluid exchange during sleep provide improved quality of life for the patients. Continuous flow PD (CFPD) through potential application of sorbents is also under intensive research.

However, long-term PD is associated with progressive loss of UF capacity, resulting in ultimate discontinuation of PD. This is related to the inflammation, new vessel formation (neoangiogenesis) and fibrotic thickening of the peritoneal membrane (PM). Bio-incompatible PD fluid, along with peritonitis, is the major contributor to the PM change. IL-6, VEGF, TGF-β, connective tissue growth factor (CTGF) are suspected as mediators of the PM injury. There has been recent development of newer biocompatible fluids characterized by neutral pH, non-glucose or low GDP content. Further research will follow in order to develop a more biocompatible PD fluid.

Chapter IV - Because renal interstitial fibrosis occurs in virtually all the progressive renal diseases leading to end-stage renal failure controlling it would be a reasonable therapeutic strategy. Plasminogen activator inhibitor-1 (PAI-1) is the main regulator of plasminogen activator-plasmin system and is attracting attention as one of the key molecules in the development of renal fibrosis. It is weakly expressed in normal kidney, but its expression is upregulated in various renal diseases leading to renal fibrosis. The authors have shown in mice with unilateral ureteral obstruction, a model for progressive renal interstitial fibrosis, that genetically engineered mice deficient for PAI-1 develop less renal fibrosis than wild-type mice. The authors have also shown in spontaneously hypercholesterolemic rat, a model of chronic progressive renal disease with massive proteinuria, that drugs reported to inhibit PAI-1 *in vitro*, such as angiotensin II type-1 receptor blocker and peroxisome proliferator-activated receptor gamma (PPAR-γ) agonist, inhibit renal PAI-1 expression and have a significant renoprotective effect. PAI-1 is therefore a promising therapeutic target for chronic progressive renal disease.

This chapter describes the evidence for the important role of PAI-1 and the value of therapeutic approaches targeting PAI-1 in progressive renal fibrosis.

Chapter V - Acute poststreptococcal glomerulonephritis (APSGN) develops as an acute nephritic syndrome 1–3 weeks after a streptococcal infection and usually heals without progression. One of the few types of human glomerulonephritis with a clearly defined course of events, it is therefore the appropriate type for which to analyze the process of glomerular injury and resolution. The histological hallmark of this disease in light microscopy is prominent glomerular endocapillary proliferation and in immunofluorescence is granular C3 and/or IgG deposition on the capillary wall. The pathogenic mechanism of APSGN has thus been described by an immune complex theory that involves glomerular deposition of nephritogenic streptococcal antigen and subsequent formation of immune complexes *in situ* and/or the deposition of circulating antigen-antibody complexes. Glomerular immunoglobulin deposition, however, is not often prominent in this disease and the site of glomerular cell infiltration is not the site of immune complex deposition: the major site of inflammation is the inner side of the glomerular tufts, while in early phase of this disease the immune complex is on the outer side of the glomerular tufts. How the nephritogenic antigen induces the glomerular manifestation of APSGN is unknown, and the identity of the causative antigen remains a matter of debate. The authors recently isolated and characterized a novel nephritogenic antigen of APSGN that The authors call the nephritis-associated plasmin receptor (NAPlr). It is identical to the plasmin receptor for group A streptococcus and can stabilize and protect plasmin activity from inhibitors *in vitro*. Glomerular NAPlr deposits are present in essentially all patients with early-phase APSGN. The localization of NAPlr differs from that of C3 or IgG but is almost identical to that of plasmin activity. NAPlr thus has a direct non-immunologic function as a plasmin receptor and might contribute to the pathogenesis of APSGN by maintaining proteolytic activity. Analysis of glomerular hypercellularity revealed that most of the infiltrating cells are macrophages (MΦs) and neutrophils and that a few are CD4+, CD45RO+ T cells. There is a significant positive correlation between the numbers of glomerular infiltrating CD4+ T cells and MΦs. They have also found prominent resident glomerular cell proliferation, particularly in the early phase of APSGN. These histological features suggest that an antigen-specific event related to delayed-type hypersensitivity is involved in the development of APSGN. The authors found prominent glomerular cell apoptosis in the early phase of APSGN. The numbers of both proliferating and apoptotic cells decrease exponentially over time, but the decrease is more pronounced for proliferating cells. Thus, apoptosis is predominant in the later phase of the disease and might contribute to the decrease in the number of glomerular cells.

In this chapter their proposed mechanisms of the development and resolution of APSGN are described with special attention to the characteristics of the recently isolated nephritogenic antigen and the contributions of plasmin activity, cell mediated immunity, and apoptosis.

Chapter VI - Autosomal Dominant Polycystic Kidney Disease (ADPKD) is the cause of renal failure in 5-10% of the patients in dialysis or transplantation. Several conditions are associated to the rate of progression. In this manuscript the authors presented data on the rate of progression of a large cohort of patients followed in a single institution by a one and only nephrologist for a mean time of 95 months.

Methods: 420 patients (178 males; 360 with a positive family history) were regularly seen in outpatient setting since 1989, the mean follow-up was 95,0 ± 64,4 months [median 85, range 2-353] and the mean number of visits was 15,4 ± 11,3 [median 12, range 1-55 visits]. In each visit analysis of the renal function, blood pressure and relevant clinical data were registered. The rate of progression to chronic renal failure (CRF) was evaluated using Kaplan-Meier (KM) survival analysis. Additionally the authors compared the slope of the regression line of the 1/serum creatinine versus time plot (PLOT) as well as the rate of deterioration of creatinine clearance, calculated by Cockroft-Gault formula (CGF), in 226 patients with a minimum follow-up of 60 months and 6 visits.

Results: Mean age of renal death was 56,1 ± 11,9 years in men as compared to 57,8 ± 12,7 in women (p=ns); KM survival curves showed that 50% of the men started dialysis by the age of 65,8 while women started at 69,8 years (95% CI: 62,1-69,4; log rank 2,88; p=0,08). Similarly, no differences were found between patients who inherited the disease from their father and those who inherited from their mothers. Patients with mean office blood pressure (MAP) higher than 106 had worse renal prognosis (log-rank 4,2; p<0,04). Patients who had haematuria (p<0,001) or who had any urologic symptoms (haematuria, renal colic or cyst infection) had considerably worse prognosis than those whose follow-up was uneventful (p<0,02). As ascertained by the slope of PLOT, patients with fast progression (slope < –0,0043), more had initiated dialysis (p<0,001), had more haematuria (p<0,001), higher MAP (p<0,001) and a higher rate of deterioration of CGF (p<0,001) than those with slow progression (slope > 0,001). Similarly, patients with CGF rate greater than 4,27 ml/min/year (fast progressors) are older, more had started dialysis, had more haematuria, higher MAP and steeper slope in the PLOT analysis.

Conclusions: ADPKD patients with urologic symptoms and higher blood pressure had increased risk for progression to CRF.

Chapter VII - Chronic kidney disease (CKD) often clusters within families. Studies have suggested possible links between CKD and a variety of alterations or polymorphisms of candidate genes coding for putative mediators, including the renin angiotensin aldosterone system (RAAS), nitric oxide synthetase, kallikrein, interleukin 1, tumour necrosis factor α and other cytokines, growth factors such as platelet derived growth factor and transforming growth factor β, plasminogen activator inhibitor, complement factors and immunoglobulins.

On the one hand, only between 30–40% with diabetes type I and 10–20% of type II diabetics will develop nephropathy. On the other hand nephropathy may develop in some patients despite excellent blood sugar control, but it may fail to develop in others despite long-term hyperglycemia. Clinically one can apply the rule that the presence of retinopathy makes it more likely that nephropathy will also develop, whereas in patients who have had a history of 20 years of diabetes without renal involvement the occurrence of significant diabetic nephropathy is unlikely. These findings suggest that apart from the actual blood sugar control there are hereditary and environmental factors contributing to the development of diabetic nephropathy. The prevalence of nephropathy among diabetics is variable in different ethnic groups such that it is relatively increased in African Americans, Native Americans, Mexican Americans, Polynesians, Australian Aborigines and urbanized Indo-Asian immigrants to the United Kingdom when compared to Caucasians. Apart from the genetic make-up, social factors such as the accessibility of health care certainly play a role in some of these populations.

In the development of arterial hypertension the influence of nutritional and environmental factors is paramount, as illustrated by the results of the Intersalt study. Disease progression correlates positively with weight gain, alcohol consumption, and to some degree salt intake.

There are genetic factors involved though, which is obvious looking at familial clustering, 70% of hypertensive patients have a positive family history. Monozygotic twins will more often have parallel development of hypertension as compared with heterozygote twins. There are genetically defined populations with significantly increased hypertension incidence, such as Afro-Americans in the US. Investigations in patients with essential hypertension showed links to various candidate genes, such as angiotensinogen, adducin (which is part of the cytoskeleton and involved in salt reabsorption), the beta-adrenergous receptor and several other genes coding for subunits of the epithelial sodium channel (ENaC).

Some genetic tubular disorders are also associated with hypertension.

Hippocrates is believed to have coined the sentence: It is more important to know *who* has a disease, than to know what disease someone has. That shows that pharmacotherapy being as individualized as possible has been regarded as an ideal since ancient times—especially since "the dosage makes the poison", as Paracelsus pointed out, i.e. adverse effects can easily obscure the healing success. With some justification the concept of pharmacogenetics may be described as the scientific quintessence of these two ancient medical sayings: the individual response to any medicine is influenced by the genetic makeup of the patient which therefore should be taken into consideration before dosing.

In principle, genetic factors can interfere in two ways with pharmacotherapy— with pharmacokinetics (i.e. achieving sufficient concentrations of the active compound at the site of action) and with pharmacodynamics (i.e. the interaction of the active compound with its receptor). An example for the former is the cytochrome P450 enzymes, or the MDR1/ABCB1 gene product, a transport protein which forms an absorption barrier by carrying various compounds back into the intestinal lumen (efflux pump, related to the SLC uptake transporter). Examples for the latter would be the polymorphisms of the calcimimetic receptor and the angiotensin receptors.

Chapter VIII - Therapeutic plasma exchanges (TPE) have been firstly performed with centrifugation devices used in blood banking procedures. Nowadays TPE are increasingly performed in intensive nephrology care units using hemodialysis generators and membrane plasma separation that ensures better efficiency and simplicity. However, prescription in different medical pathologies often depends on weak evidence-based recommendations and is guided by clinician's own experience. In this review, after recalling rationale of plasmapheresis prescription, the authors will discuss evidence level of most common indications of TPE in nephrology. Currently, strongest evidence-based data have found that benefit of TPE is demonstrated in diseases like haemolytic uremic syndrome, anti-glomerular basement membrane nephropathy and humoral renal allograft rejection. But this benefit is still controversed in ANCA-associated vasculitis and clearly absent in lupus nephritis. More randomized clinical trials are needed.

Chapter IX - Macrophages have classically been recognized as active players that mediate and promote renal fibrosis. However, several recent studies including ours have suggested a beneficial anti-fibrotic role of infiltrating macrophages in some settings of obstructive nephropathy. Furthermore, recent investigations indicating that macrophages can be functionally distinguished into two broad phenotypes, and that macrophages play a role in both inflammation and repair during the process of inflammatory responses, has superseded the classical injurious view of macrophages. As a result, the exact role of interstitial macrophages upon various facets of renal fibrosis has emerged as an important challenge that needs to be addressed. In this chapter, the authors focus upon the potentially anti-fibrotic actions of infiltrating macrophages in obstructive nephropathy and discuss the potential mechanisms that may regulate the effect of macrophages upon renal interstitial fibrosis.

Chapter X - Two decades have passed since the first reports were published proposing that risk for diabetic nephropathy may be genetically determined. Since then, efforts using the candidate gene approach and conventional genome linkage scans have met with limited success. The feasibility of performing genome wide association studies (GWAS) has been realized in recent years and results from these on diabetic nephropathy will soon be available.

These studies will undoubtedly throw light on the involvement of novel genes in the pathogenesis of this complication. Nevertheless, it is also expected on the basis of the collective GWAS experience so far that these genes will have limited effect sizes (ORs typically <1.4). Furthermore, these genes will account for a very small proportion of the genetic risk. Importantly, it is quite unlikely that they are responsible for the linkage signals that have been observed in specific chromosomal regions of the human genome. Sieving the wheat consisting of both major genes purportedly lying in the linkage regions as well as additional minor genes from the chaff will continue to be challenging.

In: Nephrology – Dialysis - Transplantation
Editors: Endre Kruger and Kelemen Hahn

ISBN 978-1-60741-736-1
© 2009 Nova Science Publishers, Inc.

Chapter I

New Pathogenic Perspectives in Diabetic Renal Disease: Diabetic Nephropathy as an Inflammatory Condition

Juan F. Navarro-González**, *Carmen Mora-Fernández, Mercedes Muros and Javier García

Nephrology Service, Clinical Biochemistry Service, and Research Unit,
University Hospital Nuestra Señora de Candelaria,
Santa Cruz de Tenerife, Spain.

Abstract

Diabetes mellitus and diabetic complications have become a major public health problem. One of the most relevant diabetic complications is diabetic nephropathy, which is nowdays the main cause of end-stage renal failure and the leading cause for entry in renal replacement therapy programs. In addition, diabetic nephropathy is associated with a dramatic increase in cardiovascular risk. In spite of the improvement in our knowledge on different aspects of diabetes mellitus, the intimate mechanisms involved in the development and progression of diabetic renal injury are not yet fully known. There is now growing evidence that activation of innate immunity and the subsequent development of a chronic low grade inflammatory reaction are relevant factors in the pathogenesis of diabetes and its complications. There are diverse inflammatory cells, mediators and pathways involved in this scenario, including monocytes/macrophages, lymphocytes, neutrophils, toll-like receptors, chemoattractant cytokines, cell adhesion molecules, and pro-inflammatory cytokines. These factors play a critical role in the development of microvascular diabetic complications, including diabetic nephropathy. This chapter reviews and discusses the pathophysiological implications of inflammation in the pathogenesis of diabetic nephropathy.

* Correspondence: Juan F. Navarro-González,MD,PhD,FASN, Nephrology Service, Univerisity Hospital Nuestra Señora de Candelaria, 38010 Santa Cruz de Tenerife, Spain. E-mail: jnavgon@gobiernodecanarias.org

Introduction

The number of people with diabetes, mainly type 2, is increasing worldwide due to several reasons, including population growth, aging, urbanization, and increasing prevalence of obesity and physical inactivity. In a recent study, Wild et al. [1] showed that the number of people with diabetes in the world is expected to approximately double between 2000 and 2030, based solely upon demographic changes and assuming that age-specific prevalence remains constant. Estimations indicate that the global diabetes prevalence among adults ≥ 20 years of age would rise from around 170 million in 2000 to more than 320 million in 2030, with much of this increase occurring in developing countries. Importantly, the authors suggest that these projections might be even underestimated. They considered that even if the prevalence of obesity remains stable until 2030, which seems unlikely, it is anticipated that the number of people with diabetes will be more than double as a consequence of population aging and urbanization. However, in the light of the observed increase in prevalence of obesity in many countries of the world and the importance of obesity as a risk factor for diabetes, the number of cases of diabetes in 2030 may be considerably higher than stated in that study.

Chronic diabetes-related complications are frequent and severe, leading to handicaps and increased morbidity and mortality for the patients and a heavy financial burden for society. Much of the burden of diabetes is due to the development of vascular complications. In association with increasing diabetes prevalence, this will inevitably result in increasing proportions of deaths, mainly from cardiovascular disease, as well as increased prevalence and associated consequences of other complications of diabetes. Regarding mortality, projections for 2030 indicates that DM will be the 7th cause of death in the world, and the 4th in the high-income countries [2].

Concerning diabetic retinopathy, one of the main causes of blindness worldwide, since the early 1980's there have been studies of the variability of this complications in populations around the world and subpopulations in the United States which have demonstrated the high prevalences and incidences of this condition [3]. Using published prevalence data of diabetic retinopathy, vision-threatening diabetic retinopathy, glaucoma and cataracts from the National Health Interview Survey and the US Census Bureau, Saaddine et al. [4] have projected in a very recent study that the number of Americans 40 years or older with diabetic retinopathy and vision-threatening diabetic retinopathy will triple in 2050, from 5.5 million in 2005 to 16 million for diabetic retinopathy and from 1.2 million in 2005 to 3.4 million for vision-threatening diabetic retinopathy. Likewise, the number of cataracts will likely increase 235% by 2050. Another important diabetic complication is the diabetic foot, which remains a major medical, social and economic problem [5]. Diabetes is the major cause of non-traumatic amputation in most western countries; rates are as much as 15 times higher than in the non-diabetic population [6]. It has been estimated that up to 25% of diabetic patients will develop a foot ulcer sometime during their lives and up to 2% of patients may already have undergone amputation [7].

Finally, the present chapter will be focused in diabetic nephropathy (DN) (with special reference to this complication in type 2 diabetes), a devasting disorder that is now the leading cause of end-stage renal failure worldwide. As the epidemic of diabetes spreads so does the number of patients at risk for developing this complication, which occurs in 20% to 40% of all diabetic patients [8]. End-stage renal disease in diabetic patients, especially type 2 diabetes, is a problem of dramatically increasing importance, which has been referred to as a true epidemic [9,10]. It constitutes a medical catastrophe, not only because of the heavy strains it puts on health budgets and logistics of medical care, but also because of the immense human suffering [11]. DN accounting for approximately one third of all cases of end-stage renal disease worldwide, although in some areas such as USA or Canary Islands, it is responsible for nearly half of all new end-stage renal disease cases [12,13].

Innate Immunity, Inflammation and Diabetes Mellitus: The Change in the Paradigm

Several lines of evidence, especially in the last 15 years, have supported the hypothesis that inflammation plays a significant role in the pathogenesis of glucose disorders in adults:

1) T cell abnormalities are believed to be the major cause of autoimmune disease in type 1 diabetes, leading to the destruction of pancreatic islets. In addition, recent investigations suggest that the innate immune system plays a key role in promoting the response of autoreactive T cells triggering type 1 diabetes [14]. In type 2 diabetes, inflammation and activation of monocytes are postulated to be important for enhancing insulin resistance and may contribute to the loss of insulin secretory function by islet cells. Thus, the presence of markers of autoimmune inflammation against the pancreatic β-cell are present in cases of of non-obese adults without antecedent glucose abnormalities that develop diabetes [15,16].
2) Cross-sectional studies have shown that markers of inflammation are elevated in patients with impaired glucose tolerance and diabetes compared with subjects without these alterations [17-21].
3) An important body of evidence is derived from prospective studies, including the Atherosclerosis Risk in Communities Study [22,23], the U.S. Women's Health Study [24], the U.S. Insulin Resistance and Atherosclerosis Study [25], the European Prospective Investigation into Cancer and Nutrition (EPIC)-Postdam Study [26], the Nurses' Health Study [27], or the KORA Augsburg Study [28], which have demonstrated that different inflammatory biomarkers are strongly associated with the risk of developing prediabetic conditions as well as type 2 diabetes.
4) The study of immune gene abnormalities in animal models, although do not allow obtain firm conclusions concerning the pathogenesis of human diabetes, they can provide the necessary proof of principle. Disruption or transgenic overexpression of different immune/inflammatory genes (including tumor necrosis factor-α (TNF(α) and TNFα receptors, interleukin-6 (IL-6), intercellular adhesion molecule-1 (ICAM-1), plasminogen activator inhibitor-1, CD11b, or inducible nitric oxide synthase) in mice have a major effect on the risk of developing insulin resistance or diabetes [29-34].

5) In the last years, an increasing number of studies have reported that immune/inflammtory gene variants in humans are associated either with higher diabetes risk or with protection from diabetes. Thus, alleles in HLA loci and in the genes encoding TNFα, IL-1 receptor, IL-6, IL-6 receptor, IL-21, and CRP have been reported to be associated with type 2 diabetes [35-44].
6) Finally, interesting data have been obtained from studies showing that modulation of immune activation and inflammation by lifestyle changes as well as pharmacological interventions may modify the risk of diabetes. Data from the Finish Diabetes Prevention Study demonstrated that non-pharmacological intervention focussing on diet and physical activity resulted in attenuation of subclinical inflammation associated with a decrease in the risk of diabetes development [45]. In the West of Scotland Coronary Prevention Study [46], pravastatin administration resulted in a 30% reduction in the risk of developing type 2 diabetes, which may be related to anti-inflammatory effects, including inhibition of cytokines release by up-regulating peroxisome proliferator-activated receptor (PPAR)-α and -γ and inhibiting the NF-κB pathway) [47,48]. Likewise, several studies with thiazolidinediones, drugs with significant anti-inflammatory effects, such as inhibition of cytokine production, macrophage activation, and reduction of the levels of inflammatory markers [49-51], have reported a significant improvement in insulin sensitivity [52] and a decrease in the risk of progression to diabetes in subjects with a known high risk for developing this disease [53].

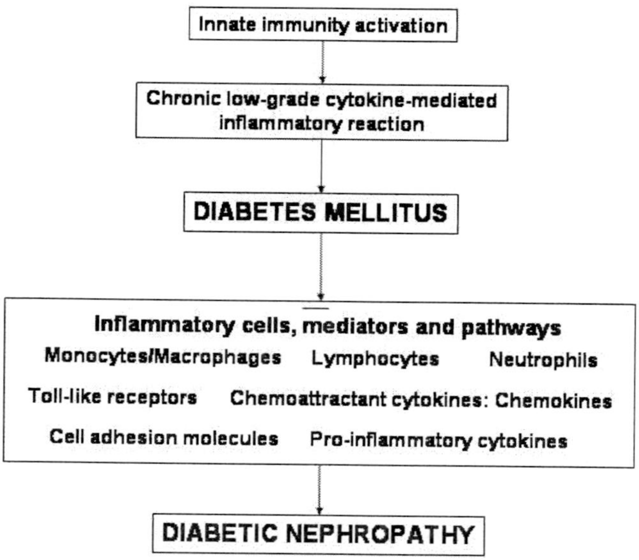

Figure 1. Schematic view of inflammatory pathogenic implications in diabetic nephropathy.

Overall, these data support the hypothesis, first proposed in 1997 and 1998 [54,55], that a widespread activation of the innate immune system and a subsequent ongoing cytokine-induced acute-phase response (low-grade inflammation) is closely involved in the pathogenesis of type 2 diabetes (Figure 1) [56]. Several factors have been proposed as potential mechanisms of activated innate immunity, including age, genetics and race, fetal and neonatal programming, cytokines (IL-1β, IL-6, TNFα), dietary factors, smoking, and stress [56].

Innate Immunity, Inflammation and Diabetic Complications

Complications of diabetes affect many tissues and organs, causing retinopathy, nephropathy, neuropathy, cardiovascular diseases, peripheral vascular disease, stroke, and periodontal pathologies. The realization that abnormalities in innate immunity participate in the pathogenesis of diabetes, and that diabetes is a proinflammatory cytokine-associated disease, lead to question whether innate immunity and inflammation are also pathogenic factors in the development of diabetic complications (Table 1) [57].

Table 1. Innate immunity and inflammatory factors involved in the pathogenesis of diabetes mellitus and diabetic complications

Inflammatory cells
Monocytes, macrophages, lymphocytes, neutrophils
Toll-like receptors
Chemokines
Monocyte chemoatrractant protein-1
Fractalkine
Regulated upon activation, normal T cell expressed and secreted
Cell-adhesion molecules
Intercellular adhesion molecule-1
Vascular cell adhesion molecule -1
E-selectine
Alpha-actinin-4
Pro-inflammatory cytokines
Interleukins 1, 6, 18
Tumor necrosis factor-α

Diabetic Neuropathy

The etiology of diabetic neuropathy is complex and multifactorial. Hyperglicemia induces local metabolic, enzymatic and microvascular changes, with a relevant role of inflammatory pathways [58]. Changes induced by chronic hyperglicaemia lead to dysregulation of pro-inflammatory cytokines. These molecules are produced locally by resident and infiltrating cells. These molecules have important effects on homeostasis of glia and neurons in central, peripheral and autonomic nervous system [59]. It has been demonstrated that endogenous TNF-α production is accelerated in microvascular and neural tissues, which may undergo an increased microvascular permeability, hypercoagulability, and nerve damage, thus initiating and promoting the development of characteristics lesions of diabetic neuropathy [60].

Diabetic Retinopathy

There is an accumulating body of evidence that immunological mechanisms play a prominent role in the pathogenesis of diabetic retinopathy, which is characterized by many features typical of inflammation [61,62]. The upregulation of cytokines and other inflammatory mediators leading to persistent low-grade inflammation and an influx of leukocytes, is believed to contribute actively to diabetic retinopathy-associated damage to the retinal vasculature and retinal neovascularization [63].

Experimental animal investigations have shown that mRNA expression of pro-inflammatory transcription factors, such as NF-κB [63], as well as inflammatory cytokines, including IL-1 and TNF-α, is increased in the retina early in the course of diabetes [64,65]. In addition, inhibition of these inflammatory molecules has demonstrated beneficial effects in the prevention of early diabetic retinopathy [66]. Regarding clinical studies, these investigations have shown elevated levels of pro-inflammatory cytokines in the vitreous fluid of patients with proliferative diabetic retinopathy, which are related with activity and progression of retinal injury [67,68].

Diabetic Nephropathy

Initially thought that renal injury in DN is mainly caused by metabolic (secondary to hyperglycemia) and hemodynamic alterations (such as hyperfiltration and hyperperfusion). Specific metabolically driven glucose dependent pathways are activated within DN. These pathways induce oxidative stress, polyol pathway flux, hexosamine flux and accumulation of advanced glycated end-products in the kidney [69]. Hemodynamic factors are further influencing the pathogenesis of DN and include elevations of systemic and intra-glomerular pressure and activation of vasoactive hormones including renin-angiotensin-aldosterone system, endothelin and urotensin. These altered hemodynamics act independently, and in concert with metabolic pathways to activate intracellular second messengers [70]. However, there is now clear evidence that the pathogenesis of DN is multifactorial and is comprised of genetic and environmental factors activating a multitude of intra- and extra-renal pathways, where metabolic and hemodynamic changes are only one aspect of a complex series of pathophysiological alterations [71,72]. The last few years have provided a better insight into the complex pathophysiology of DN on a molecular level, and therefore, we now know that inflammatory molecules, mediators and pathways are determinants in the development and progression of renal injury in diabetes mellitus.

Table 2. Potential pathophysiologic mechanisms of inflammation-mediated renal injury in diabetes mellitus

- Production of reactive oxygen species, cytokines and proteases
- Interferon-γ secretion and induction of oxidative stress
- Attachment (sticking) of leukocytes, monocytes and macrophages to the endothelium and the subsequent transendothelial transmigration
- Increment of vascular endothelial permeability and proliferation of mesangial cells and matrix synthesis
- Induction of intraglomerular hemodynamic abnormalities related to prostaglandin synthesis by mesangial cells
- Induction of hemodynamic disbalance between vasodilator and vasoconstrictive mediators
- Stimulation of mesangial cell proliferation and fibronectin expression
- Alteration of extracellular matrix dynamics at both mesangial and podocyte levels
- Increment of adhesion molecules expression on endothelial and vascular smooth muscle cells
- Local activation of the local renin-angiotensin system
- Enhancement of TGF-ß signaling *via* modulation of TGF-ß receptor trafficking
- Stimulation of Th1 lymphocyte response by induction of interferon-γ production
- Modulation of natural killer cells activity
- Stimulation of proinflammatory cytokine synthesis by macrophages
- Upregulation of adhesion molecules expression
- Induction of nitric oxide production
- Stimulation of the local generation of reactive oxygen species, with alteration of the barrier function of the glomerular capillary wall
- Contribution to tubular sodium retention, glomerular volume and renal hypertrophy
- Induction of cell contraction
- Inhibition of endothelium-dependent relaxation
- Reduction of glomerular blood flow and glomerular filtration rate
- Increment of albumin permeability
- Stimulation of plasminogen-activator inhibitor type-1 tissue factor production
- Downregulation of tissue factor pathway inhibitor mRNA
- Reduction of thrombomodulin expression
- Induction of major histocompatibility complex antigen expression
- Proliferation, cytotoxicity and regulation of cell death related genes
- Induction of apoptosis

Diabetic Nephropahty Is an Inflammatory Condition: Cells, Mediators and Pathways

Results from numerous experimental and clinical studies support nowadays the concept that DN can be viewed as an inflammatory disease triggered by disordered metabolism [73]. This new conception of DN is very important from a pathogenic point of view, but more relevant, it may be transcendental from a therapeutic perspective. New targets (inflammatory molecules, inflammatory mediators, and inflammatory pathways) are described as factors involved in DN, and support the rationale for the blockade of inflammatory mechanisms. This may lead to new therapeutic approaches that can be fully translated into clinical treatments, and therefore, hopes for better strategies to reduce the burden of DN may be realized.

Cells: Macrophages, Lymphocytes and Neutrophils

Early studies suggested that immune cells might be involved in the development and progression of DN. Nowadays, there is no doubt that immune cells participate in the vascular injury in the conditions of DN, and their migration into the kidney is a crucial step in the progression of this complication [74].

Macrophage accumulation is a feature of type 2 diabetes and is associated with the development of diabetic complications (nephropathy, atherosclerosis, neuropathy and retinopathy) whereas macrophage-depletion studies in rodent models have demonstrated a causal role for these cells in the development of diabetic complications [75,76]. Diverse components of the diabetic milieu, such as high glucose, advanced glycation end-products or oxidized low-density lipoproteins, promote macrophage accumulation (via induction of chemokines and adhesion molecules) and activation within diabetic tissues. Macrophages mediate diabetic injury through a variety of mechanisms, including production of reactive oxygen species, cytokines and proteases, which result in tissue damage leading to sclerosis. Macrophages are one of the central mediators of renal vascular inflammation, and their accumulation is a characteristic feature of DN [77-80]. Infiltrated macrophages are found within renal diabetic tissues, and recent studies demonstrated that macrophage-derived products can induce further inflammation in the diabetic kidney [77-80].

Activated T lymphocytes have been associated with DN [81,82]. It has been suggested that the interaction between lymphocyte function-associated antigen-1, which is constitutively expressed by naïve as well as effector T cells, and ICAM-1, which is expressed by renal endothelial, epithelial, and mesangial cells [83-85], play a significant role during T cell migration into kidney. Indeed, homing of CD4-T cells into glomeruli of diabetic kidney was decreased in ICAM-1-deficient-db/db mice compared with wild type db/db mice [86]. In addition, the activation of CD4- and CD8-T cells by AGEs can initiate IFN-γ secretion by T cells [87], which will induce further inflammation and oxidative stress within renal tissues.

Finally, the activated status of blood neutrophils is one of the most striking features of leukocytes from patients with diabetes [88,89]. DN neutrophils exhibited an elevated expression of CD11b [88], which could play a role in the directing of neutrophil migration in the renal inflamed tissues expressing upregulated levels of ICAM-1. In addition, spontaneous adhesion of neutrophils from patients with diabetes is increased significantly compared with adhesion of neutrophils from patients with normoalbuminuria as well as healthy control subjects [89].

Toll-Like Receptors

In 1997, vertebrate homologs of the *Drosophila* spp. transmembrane PRR 'Toll' were identified and termed the 'Toll-like receptors' (TLRs). TLRs are a family of evolutionarily conserved receptors that are named for their genetic similarity to receptors found in *Drosophila melanogaster* [90]. To date, 11 human TLRs have been cloned.

TLRs are transmembrane proteins which have a leucine-rich extracellular domain and a conserved cytoplasmic domain [91], which is homologous to the IL-1 and IL-18 receptors, called the Toll/IL-1 receptor homology (TIR) domain [92]. TLR and IL-1 receptor family members may signal through the use of an analogous framework of signaling molecules [93]. Signaling through the TLRs stimulates the production of reactive oxygen and nitrogen-intermediate molecules, cytokines, chemokines, adhesion molecules, and acute phase proteins [91,94].

Each TLR activates a number of signalling pathways, some of which are common to all TLRs and some of which are specific to particular TLR types. This differential induction pattern is dependent largely on which cytoplasmic adaptor molecules are present to associate with the intracytoplasmic domain of the TLRs [95]. These adaptors, which all contain TIR domains, include MyD88 (myeloid differentiation primary response protein), TIRAP (TIR domain-containing adaptor protein), TRIF (TIR-domain-containing adaptor inducing interferon β), and TRAM (TRIF-related adaptor molecule) [96].

TLRs recognition of self-ligands may be involved in pathologic inflammatory states because they are able to recognize endogenous ligands such as heat shock proteins 60, 70, and 96, extra domain A-containing fibronectin fragments, hyaluronan fragments, fibrinogen, β-defensins, oxidized low-density lipoprotein, and heparan sulfate [93]. The interaction and modulation of cytokine release has caused the TLRs to be investigated for their role in rheumatoid arthritis, Crohn's disease, ulcerative colitis, psoriasis, chronic obstructive pulmonary disease, and atherosclerosis, as well as in diabetes mellitus [93,97].

The basic mechanism of danger recognition via TLR signalling in response to exogenous and endogenous ligands, as well as cellular damage may also be involved in renal disease. Initial studies suggest that several TLRs, such as TLR2 and TLR4, can induce chemokine expression in tubular epithelial cells, and that TLR9 is expressed on infiltrating antigen-presenting cells during immune injury. TLR-mediated immune activation may occur during any type of renal injury by exposure to an increasing number of exogenous or endogenous molecules, and it has been implicated in diverse renal diseases, including immunecomplex glomerulonephritis, allograft rejection, acute renal injury, lupus nephritis or vasculitis [98-102].

Chemoattractant Cytokines: Chemokines

The migration of leukocytes into extravascular tissues involves a cascade of molecular events, including the elaboration of chemotactic factors and chemokines, the response to these factors, the interaction of leukocytes with endothelial cells, and leukocyte transmigration through the blood vessel wall [103-106]. Chemokines and chemokine receptors are key elements involved in inflammatory cell interactions and recruitment. Expression of inflammatory chemokines can be elicited by almost any stimulus that alters cellular homeostasis, such as infections and immune disorders [107]. However, inappropriately elevated expression of inflammatory chemokines may result in extensive tissue damage caused by activated leukocytes [108,109]. Differential expression of chemokines and their receptors provides the molecular mechanisms that lead to the precise coordination of inflammatory cell migration in renal inflammatory diseases [110]. The diabetic kidney comprises a great and complex pathophysiological network of interrelate actions, no yet fully known, although there is growing evidence supporting the role of chemokines and their receptors in the pathogenesis of DN [111].

Monocyte Chemoattractant Protein-1

In 1996, Rovin et al. [112] reported that biologically active monocyte chemoattractant protein-1 (MCP-1) was present in the urine of patients with various glomerular diseases, including DN, and also that the urinary levels of MCP-1 correlate with both the extent of proteinuria and the number of glomerular macrophages. Later studies confirmed these previous findings [113-116], showing that urinary MCP-1 levels also correlated with the number of CD68-positive infiltrating monocyte/macrophage cells in the interstitium [117]. Therefore, it was suggested that locally produced MCP-1 might be involved in the development of renal injury in DN, especially in the formation of tubulointerstitial lesions possibly through monocyte/macrophage recruitment and activation [118].

Recent experimental studies in diabetic mice, both streptozotocin-induced and db/db mice, which were deficient in the gene encoding MCP-1, demonstrated protection from nephropathy, with marked reductions in glomerular and interstitial macrophage accumulation, histological damage, and renal fibrosis [119,120]. These findings strongly suggest that neutralizing MCP-1 activity would be an important therapeutic goal in the treatment of DN [121]. From this perspective, a recent study using propagermanium (a MCP-1 receptor (CCR2) antagonist) showed that blockade of this pathway ameliorated glomerulosclerosis in a DN experimental model [122]. Finally, modulation of MCP-1 has been related to beneficial renoprotective effects of clinical therapeutic strategies in patients with DN, such as blockade of the rennin-angiotensin-aldosterone system. [123-125].

Fractalkine

Fractalkine/CX3CL1 is a unique chemokine that exists in membrane-bound as well as in soluble form, and therefore functions not only as a chemoattractant but also as an adhesion molecule. It is expressed on endothelial cells activated by proinflammatory cytokines, whereas the fractalkine receptor, CX3CR1, is expressed on cytotoxic effector lymphocytes and monocytes/macrophages [126,127]. Accumulating evidence has shown that fractalkine is involved in the pathogenesis of various diseases with a significant inflammatory background, including atherosclerosis, cardiovascular disease, graft rejection, glomerulonephritis, and diabetes [128-140].

Concerning DN, it has been demonstrated an increased fractalkine and CX3CR1 mRNA expression in diabetic kidneys compared with that in controls at early stages of renal injury. Fractalkine staining in diabetic kidneys was clearly detected, along with glomerular capillary lumen and peritubular capillaries. In addition, CX3CR1 positive cell infiltration in diabetic glomeruli was also found [141].

RANTES

Regulated upon activation, normal T cell expressed and secreted (RANTES), is also called CCL5 (chemokine (C-C motif) ligand 5). This chemokine was identified by subtractive hybridization screening for genes expressed by human T lymphocytes 3–5 days after activation [142]. It is a potent chemoattractant for monocytes/macrophages and granulocytes, but also for T cells, and is involved in enhanced chronic inflammation. RANTES/CCL5 is expressed by various cell types including lymphocytes, fibroblasts, mesangial cells and renal tubular epithelial cells [143-145]. The importance of RANTES in renal disease was first apparent in renal graft rejection, where rejecting grafts exhibited large amounts of RANTES bound to the vascular endothelium [146]. We now know that RANTES released from stromal cells in damaged tissues binds to glycosaminoglycans on the endothelium, where it serves as a 'signpost' for recruitment of immune cells. Expression of high levels of RANTES is associated with a wide range of renal diseases including glomerulonephrities and interstitial nephrities, as well as DN.

Elevated systemic concentrations of RANTES have been described to be higher in individuals with impaired glucose tolerance or type 2 diabetes as compared to healthy subjects, suggesting that this chemokine can be involved in the development of type 2 diabetes independent of metabolic syndrome-related risk factors [147]. In addition, the Finnish Diabetes Prevention Study showed that increased serum levels of RANTES were associated in the intervention group with progression to type 2 diabetes [148].

A strong upregulation of RANTES was observed in renal biopsies from patients with type 2 diabetes and overt nephropathy, mainly in tubular cells. In addition, the tubular expression of this chemokine was correlated with the magnitude of the proteinuria and with interstitial cell infiltration [149]. Regarding the chemokine receptor for RANTES, called CCR5, this molecule is mainly expressed by infiltrating T cells in the interstitium, but was not detected on intrinsic cells of glomerular, tubular, or vascular structures [150]. A human renal biopsy study of patients with various renal diseases showed that glomerular CCR5-positive cells were closely correlated with extracapillary lesions, while interstitial CCR5-positive cells were correlated with interstitial lesions and urinary RANTES levels [151].

Cell Adhesion Molecules

Cell adhesion molecules are proteins located on the cell surface involved with the binding with other cells or with the extracellular matrix in the process called cell adhesion.

These proteins are typically transmembrane receptors and are composed of three domains: an intracellular domain that interacts with the cytoskeleton, a transmembrane domain, and an extracellular domain that interacts either with other adhesion molecules of the same kind (homophilic binding) or with other adhesion molecules or the extracellular matrix (heterophilic binding).

Intercellular Adhesion Molecule-1 (ICAM-1) and Vascular Cell Adhesion Molecule -1 (VCAM-1)

ICAM-1 and VCAM-1 are adhesion molecules that belong to the Immunoglobulin superfamily [152,153]. ICAM-1 is continuously present in low concentrations in the membranes of leukocytes and endothelial cells. Upon cytokine stimulation, the concentrations greatly increase. It is also expressed by macrophages, and lymphocytes. When activated, leukocytes binds to endothelial cells via ICAM-1 and then transmigrates into tissues. VCAM-1 promotes the adhesion of lymphocytes, monocytes, eosinophils, and basophils, and it is primarly expressed by endothelial and smooth muscle cells.

ICAM-1 interacts with T cell and stimulates migration into the kidney. In ICAM-1-deficient-db/db mice, homing of $CD4^+$ cells into glomeruli of diabetic kidneys was decreased as compared with wild type db/db mice [86,154]. In addition, increased expression of ICAM-1 has been demonstrated in models of DN, showing a direct association with renal injury and progression [155,156]. Clinical studies have demonstrated that diabetic patients with nephropathy have elevated concentrations of ICAM-1 compared to subjects without renal injury [157,158].

Experimental studies in diabetic mice have shown an increased endothelial cell expression of VCAM-1, as well as by infiltrating cells in the renal interstitium [159]. Cross-sectional clinical studies have shown an elevation of circulating VCAM-1 in patients with DN [160-162], while clinical prospective investigations in individuals with type 2 DM have shown that patients with high plasma concentrations of soluble VCAM-1 had an increased risk of death, which was independent of major risk factors for developing elevated urinary albumin excretion, such as high blood pressure and poor glycemic control [163].

E-selectin

E-selectin, also known as CD62E, is a cell adhesion molecule expressed only on endothelial cells activated by cytokines. E-selectin recognises and binds to sialylated carbohydrates present on the surface proteins of certain leukocytes. During inflammation, E-selectin plays an important part in recruiting leukocytes to the site of injury. The local release of cytokines IL-1 and TNF by damaged cells induces the over-expression of E-selectin on endothelial cells of nearby blood vessels. Leukocytes in the blood expressing the correct ligand will bind with low affinity to E-selectin, causing the leukocytes to "roll" along the internal surface of the blood vessel as temporary interactions are made and broken [164].

Expression of E-selectin is significantly increased in the glomeruli and the interstitium of patients with DN. E-selectin is both expressed along the glomerular capillaries and the peritubular capillaries in the interstitium. E-selectin was not correlated with the number of infiltrated leukocytes in the glomeruli. However, and interestingly, the E-selectin expression on peritubular capillaries was correlated with the number of infiltrated CD14 positive cells in the interstitium [165]. Induction of E-selectin mRNA expression in glomeruli by proinflammatory stimuli is augmented in streptozotocin-induced diabetic mice as compared with control mice, while immunohistochemical analysis demonstrates that selective expression of E-selectin in glomeruli is augmented predominantly in epithelial cells, depending on the duration of diabetes mellitus [166].

Finally, from a clinical perspective, the European Diabetes (EURODIAB) Prospective Complications Study showed that soluble E-selectin levels had positive associations with albuminuria and cardiovascular disease [167]. More recently, data from the Diabetes Control and Complications Trial (DCCT)/Epidemiology of Diabetes Intervention and Complications (EDIC) cohort have demonstrated that soluble E-selectin shows strong evidence for an association with nephropathy, even after correction for conventional risk factors (total and HDL cholesterol, smoking, age, sex, glycated hemoglobin, blood pressure, and waist-to-hip ratio), and duration of diabetes [168].

Alpha-Actinin-4

Alpha actinins belong to the spectrin gene superfamily which represents a diverse group of cytoskeletal proteins. Alpha-actinin-4 is not an adhesion molecule; it is an actin filament crosslinking protein that interacts with intercellular adhesion molecules. The expression of alpha-actinin-4 has been identified on cultured mouse podocytes, being suggested that it is an essential component of the glomerular filtration barrier [169,170]. Alpha-actinin-4 interacts with integrins and strengthens the podocyte-GBM interaction thereby stabilizing glomerular architecture and preventing disease [171].

In a recent study, Kimura et al. [172] examined alpha-actinin-4 expression in the glomerulus using kidney specimens from patients with DN. They demonstrated at both mRNA and protein levels (by in situ hybridization and immunohistochemistry) that alpha-actinin-4 were exclusively expressed on podocytes. Interestingly, renal samples from patients with moderate mesangial expansion group (who showed greater proteinuria and more advanced glomerular changes than those with mild mesangial expansion group and the control) exhibited reduced alpha-actinin-4 expression for both mRNA and protein. The percentage of cells positive for alpha-actinin-4 mRNA and area positive for the protein were correlated inversely with glomerular mesangial expansion and 24-hour urinary protein excretion, suggesting that down-regulation of alpha-actinin-4 mRNA and protein expression may relate to severity of DN.

Pro-Inflammatory Cytokines

Cytokines are a group of pharmacologically active low molecular weight polypeptides produced widely throughout the body by cells of diverse embryological origin, that possess autocrine, paracrine and juxtacrine effects. These molecules are relevant humoral mediators in a highly complex coordinate network regulating inflammatory and immune responses; in addition, they exert important pleiotropic actions and are cardinal effectors of the inflammatory and immune system [173-175]. A set of features characterize cytokines, including: 1) constitutive production usually low or absent; 2) production is transient, with the action radius usually short, and regulated by various inducing stimuli at the level of transcription or translation; 3) cytokines actions are mediated by binding to high affinity cell surface receptors, and these actions can be attributed to an altered pattern of gene expression in the target cells; 4) from a phenotipic perspective, cytokine effects lead to a variation in the rate of cell proliferation, change and cell differentiation state and/or change in the expression of some differentiated functions; 5) cytokines often have multiple target cells and multiple actions, and different cytokines may have an overlapping spectrum of actions; 6) exposure of cells to various cytokines at a time may lead to qualitatively different responses; and 7) there are complex interrelationships among these molecules: a cytokine may alter the expression of receptors for another cytokine, influence signalling by receptors for other cytokines, and influence the production of another cytokine [173-175].

Cytokines play an important role in many physiological responses, but they are also involved in the pathophysiology of a range of diseases and their complications [173]. The report that glomerular basement membranes from diabetic rats induced significantly greater levels of TNF-α and IL-1 production from cultured peritoneal macrophages than basement membranes from normal nondiabetic rats, suggested for the first time that inflammatory cytokines may participate in the pathogenesis of DN [176,177]. Later studies have demonstrated that infiltrating monocytes/macrophages and T cells, as well as intrinsic renal cells (endothelial, mesangial, glomerular, and tubular epithelial cells) are able to synthesize pro-inflammatory cytokines [178,179].

Interleukins: IL-1, IL-6, IL-18

Renal expression of IL-1 has been demonstrated to be increased in renal models of DN [180,181], which has been related to an elevated expression of chemotactic factors and adhesion molecules. Thus, IL-1 enhances ICAM-1 and VCAM-1 synthesis by glomerular endothelial cells, and induce de novo synthesis and expression of ICAM-1 by glomerular mesangial cells and renal tubular epithelial cells. In addition, this cytokine induce transient expression of E-selectin by endothelial cells [182,183]. IL-1 has been involved in the development of intraglomerular hemodynamic abnormalities related to prostaglandin synthesis by mesangial cells. Treatment of glomerular mesangial cells with recombinant human IL-1 induces prostaglandin E2 synthesis and the release of a phospholipase A2 activity [184], whereas pre-treatment of resting mesangial cells with this cytokine results in an amplified secretory prostaglandin E2 response to angiotensin II [185]. Finally, IL-1 directly increases vascular endothelial cell permeability [186] and disregulates hyaluronan generation by renal proximal tubular epithelial cells [187,188].

Analysis of kidney biopsies from patients with DN by high-resolution in situ hybridization demonstrated that mesangium, interstitium, tubules and infiltrating cells were positive for IL-6 mRNA, with a significant relationship between severity of diabetic glomerulopathy (mesangial expansion) and expression of IL-6 mRNA in glomerular cells (mesangial cells and podocytes) [189]. Clinical studies have showed that serum levels of IL-6 were significantly higher in type 2 diabetic patients with nephropathy than those observed in cases of diabetic patients without renal disease [190], with a significant association between IL-6 and glomerular basement membrane thickening, a crucial lesion of DN and a strong predictor of progression of renal disease [191,192]. Recent studies have demonstrated a significant overexpression of IL-6 in the diabetic rat kidney, with this increase in the renal cortex mRNA levels of IL-6 being directly and significantly associated with an elevation in its urinary excretion [181]. Importantly, wet kidney weight, an accurate index of renal hypertrophy and one of the earliest renal changes during diabetes [193], was increased in diabetic rats and directly associated with renal mRNA expression of IL-6, as well as with urinary excretion of this cytokine [181]. Moreover, a direct correlation was observed between urinary levels and renal expression of IL-6 with markers or renal injury (urinary albumin excretion) [181].

IL-18 is a cytokine that belongs to the IL-1 superfamily. Apart from its physiological role, IL-18 is also able to induce severe inflammatory reactions, which suggests its potential role in inflammatory disorders. IL-18 is a potent inflammatory cytokine that induces interferon-γ [194] and leads to production of other inflammatory cytokines (including IL-1 and TNF-α), upregulation of ICAM-1, as well as to apoptosis of endothelial cells [195-197]. IL-18 is constitutively expressed in renal tubular epithelia, and recent studies have demonstrated that infiltrating monocytes/macrophages and T cells, along with proximal tubular cells are potential sources of this cytokine [198-200]. Recently, serum and urinary levels of IL-18 have been reported to be increased in patients with DN, with an independent relationship between these parameters and markers of glomerular (urinary albumin excretion) and tubulo-interstitial (urinary excretion of β-2 microglobulin) injury [201-203]. In a longitudinal study, serum and urinary IL-18 concentrations were directly correlated with albumin excretion rate, as well as with changes in albuminuria during the follow-up period [202]. Moreover, elevated IL-18 has been showed as a determinant of early renal dysfunction in type 2 DM [204].

Tumor Necrosis Factor-α

TNF-α is a cytokine involved in systemic inflammation and is a member of a group of cytokines that stimulate the acute phase reaction. This pleiotropic inflammatory peptide cytokine is mainly produced by monocytes/macrophages and T cells, although it has been demonstrated that expression and synthesis of TNF-α is not limited to hematopoietic cells. Recent studies have shown that TNF-α can be stored within cells in a pre-active form, and that the TNF-α converting enzyme can rapidly increase levels of the active cytokine [205]. Accumulating data suggest a differential TNFα action regarding whether TNFα contributes to or protects from tissue damage in acute or chronic diseases. In this scenario, tissue type, precise cellular context and composition, and timing and duration of TNFα action are important parameters determining the net effect of this cytokine *in vivo*.

Experimental studies have consistently reported that TNF-α mRNA and protein levels are increased in glomerular and proximal tubule cells from diabetic rats [178,179,181,206-208]. This cytokine and its receptors family have a variety of bioactivities that may promote the development of inflammatory actions related to the development and progression of renal injury in DM [209,210]. TNF-α plays a significant role in the development of renal hypertrophy and hyperfunction, two main alterations during the initial stage of DN [207,208]. TNF-α has a stimulatory effect on sodium-dependent solute uptake in proximal tubule cells [211]. Experimental studies in diabetic rats showed an increased urinary TNF-α excretion and sodium retention, as well as renal hypertrophy, alterations which were prevented by administration of the anti-TNF-α agent TNFR:Fc, a soluble TNF-α receptor fusion protein [208,211]. On the other hand, renal cortical mRNA levels and urinary TNFα concentrations have been direct and independently correlated to urinary albumin excretion [181,206], and more importantly, microdialysis studies demonstrated a significant increase of TNFα levels in renal interstitial fluid and urine preceding the development of albuminuria, with a direct correlation between urine and renal interstitial fluid concentrations of TNF-α and urinary albumin excretion. In addition, shortly after the rise in albuminuria, urinary TNF-α concentration showed a further significant increase, suggesting a stimulatory effect for albuminuria on the production of renal TNF-α [212].

TNF-α posses a variety of other biological activities that may participate in the pathophysiology of DN. Reported actions of TNF-α on renal cells include the activation of second messenger systems, transcription factors, synthesis of cytokines, growth factors, receptors, cell adhesion molecules, enzymes involved in the synthesis of other inflammatory mediators, acute phase proteins, and major histocompatibility complex proteins [213]. TNF-α has been demonstrated to be able to induce 1) direct renal injury [209]; 2) apoptotic and necrotic cell death [214,215]; 3) alterations of intraglomerular blood flow and glomerular filtration rate due to the hemodynamic disbalance between vasoconstrictive and vasodilatory mediators [216]; 4) alterations of endothelial permeability [217]; 5) activation of NADPH oxidase via protein kinase C/phosphatidylinositol-3 kinase and mitogen-activated protein kinase pathways, leading to the local generation of reactive oxygen species [218-220].

Clinical studies have demonstrated that diabetic patients with nephropathy have higher serum and urinary concentrations of TNF-α than non-diabetic subjects as well as diabetic patients without renal involvement. Urinary TNF-α levels showed a significant rise as DN progressed, with a direct and independent association between the levels of this cytokine and clinical markers of glomerular as well as tubulointerstitial damage [201,221,222].

Conclusion

The burden of diabetes and its complications will be one of the most important health problems in the next decades. One of the most important chronic diabetes-related complications is DN: this is nowadays the main cause of end-stage renal disease and it is associated with a dramatic increase in cardiovascular risk. Protection from development and progression of diabetic kidney disease is a challenge for nephrologists.

Over the past decade, multiple studies have helped to elucidate the associations between DM, immunity and inflammation. It is now clear that innate immunity activation and low grade chronic inflammation are cardinal processes in the appearance of DM, and that the inflammatory milieu in DM contributes significantly to the development of many of the complications of this disease, including nephropathy. The relationships between this inflammatory state and the development and progression of DN involve a very complex network, with participation of diverse cells, mediators and pathways, including monocytes, macrophages, lymphocytes, toll-like receptors, chemokines, cell adhesion molecules, and pro-inflammatory cytokines.

The current treatment of DN is still suboptimal, both in preventing its development as well as in halting its progression. The improved knowledgement of the role of inflammation in DN derives from extensive experimental studies. However, from a therapeutic perspective, clinical experience regarding the inhibition of inflammatory mechanisms for treatment of this complication is very limited. A better understanding of the role of inflammatory molecules and pathways involved in the pathophysiology of DN will facilitate the development of new and improved therapeutic targets and strategies that can be translated successfully into clinical applications in terms of prevention, remission, or even regression of DN.

References

[1] Mathers CD, Loncar D. Projections of Global Mortality and Burden of Disease from 2002 to 2030. *Plos Medicine* 2006;3:e442.

[2] Wild S, Roglic G, Green A, Sicree R, King H. Global prevalence of diabetes: Estimates for the year 2000 and projections for 2030. *Diabetes Care* 2004;27:1047–1053.

[3] Klein BE. Overview of epidemiologic studies in diabetic retinopathy. *Ophthalmic Epidemiol* 2007;14:179-183.

[4] Saaddine JB, Honeycutt AA, Narayan KM, Zhang X, Klein R, Boyle JP. Projection of diabetic retinopathy and other major eye diseases among people with diabetes mellitus: United States, 2005-2050.

[5] Boulton AJM, Vileikyte L, Ragnarson-Tennvall G, Apelqvist J. The global burden of diabetic foot disease. *Lancet* 2005;366:1719-1724.

[6] Boulton AJM. The diabetic foot: grand overview, epidemiology and pathogenesis. *Diabetes Metab. Res. Rev.* 2008;24(Suppl. 1):S3-S6.

[7] Singh N, Armstrong DG, Lipsky BA. Preventing foot ulcers in patients with diabetes. *JAMA* 2005;293:217-228.

[8] Rabkin R. Diabetic nephropathy. *Clin. Cornerstone* 2003;5:1-11.

[9] Ismail N, Becker BN, Strzelczyk P, Ritz E. Renal disease and hypertension in non–insulin-dependent diabetes mellitus. *Kidney Int* 1999;55:1-8.

[10] Carretero-Dios D, Pérez-García R, Rodríguez-Benítez P, Villaverde M, Gómez-Campedrá F, Valderrabano F. Diabetes mellitus as cause of terminal renal failure. An epidemic of the 21st Century? *Nefrologia* 2001;21(Suppl. 3):83-87.

[11] Ritz E, Rychlík I, Locatelli F, Hamili S. End-Stage Renal Failure in Type 2 Diabetes: A Medical Catastrophe of Worldwide Dimensions. *Am. J. Kidney Dis*. 1999;34:795-808.

[12] Excerpts From the United States Renal Data System 2008. Annual Data Report Atlas of Chronic Kidney Disease and End-Stage Renal Disease in the United States. Incidence and prevalence. *Am. J. Kidney Dis.* 2009;53(Suppl. 1):S171-S180.

[13] Arrieta J, Castro P, Gutiérrez Ávila G, Moreno-Alía I, Sierra T, Estébanez C, Olmos AM, González R, Fernández-Renedo C, Arias M, Cotorruelo J, Martín de Francisco AL, Zurriaga O, García-Blasco MJ, Clèries M, Vela E, García- Bazaga MA, Ramos JM, Gil-Paraíso A, Sánchez-Casajús A, Unzue JJ, Purroy A, Arteaga J, Asín JL, Gorostiza G, Torralba A, Vázquez C, Registro de Insuficiencia Renal Crónica en

tratamiento sustitutivo de Aragón, Magaz A. Informe de situación de diálisis y trasplante en España, 2004. *Nefrologia* 2007;27:279-299.

[14] Zipris D. Innate immunity and its role in type 1 diabetes. *Curr. Opin. Endocrinol Diabetes Obes*. 2008;15:326-331.

[15] Tuomi T, Groop LC, Zimmet PZ, Rowley MJ, Knowles W, Mackay IR. Antibodies to glutamic acid decarboxylase reveal latent autoimmune diabetes mellitus in adults with a non-insulin-dependent onset of disease. *Diabetes* 1993;42:359–362.

[16] Pietropaolo M, Barinas-Mitchell E, Pieropaolo SL, Kuller LH, Trucco M. Evidence of islet cell autoimmunity in elderly patients with type 2 diabetes. *Diabetes* 2000;49:32–38.

[17] Pickup JC, Chusney GC, Thomas SM, Burt D. Plasma interleukin-6, tumor necrosis factor alpha and blood cytokine production in type 2 diabetes. *Life Sci.* 2000;67:291–300.

[18] Temelkova-Kurktschiev T, Henkel E, Koelher C, Karrei K, Hanefeld M. Subclinical inflammation in newly detected type II diabetes and impaired glucose tolerance. *Diabetologia* 2002;45:151.

[19] Navarro JF, Mora C, Macía M, García J. Inflammatory parameters are independently associated with urinary albumin excretion in type 2 diabetes mellitus. *Am. J. Kidney Dis.* 2003;42:53–61.

[20] Deepa R, Velmurugan K, Arvind K, Sivaram P, Sientay C, Uday S, Mohan V. Serum levels of interleukin 6, C-reactive protein, vascular cell adhesion molecule 1, and monocyte chemotactic protein 1 in relation to insulin resistance and glucose intolerance--the Chennai Urban Rural Epidemiology Study (CURES). *Metabolism* 2006;55:1232-1238.

[21] Shankar A, Li J. Positive association between high-sensitivity C-reactive protein level and diabetes mellitus among US non-Hispanic black adults. Exp Clin Endocrinol Diabetes 2008;116:455-460.

[22] Schmidt MI, Duncan BB, Sharrett AR, Lindberg G, Savage PJ, Offenbacher S, Azambuja MI, Tracey RP, Heiss G. Markers of inflammation and prediction of diabetes mellitus in adults (Atherosclerosis Risk in Communities study): a cohort study. *Lancet* 1999; 353:1649-1652.

[23] Duncan BB, Schmidt MI, Offenbacher S, Wu KK, Savage PJ, Heiss G. Factor VIII and other hemostasis variables are related to incident diabetes in adults: the Atherosclerosis Risk in Communities (ARIC) study. *Diabetes Care* 1999; 22:767–772.

[24] Pradhan AD, Manson JE, Rifai N, Buring JE, Ridker PM. C-reactive protein, interleukin 6, and risk of developing type 2 diabetes mellitus. *JAMA* 2001; 286:327–334.

[25] Festa A, D'Agostino R, Tracey RP, Haffner SM. Elevated levels of acute-phase proteins and plasminogen activator inhibitor-1 predict the development of type 2 diabetes: the Insulin Resistance Atherosclerosis Study. *Diabetes* 2002; 51:1131–1137.

[26] Spranger J, Kroke A, Möhlig M, Hoffman K, Bergman MM, Ristow M, Boeing H, Pfeiffer AFH. Inflammatory cytokines and the risk to develop type 2 diabetes: results of the prospective population-based European Prospective Investigation into Cancer and Nutrition (EPIC) Postsdam study. *Diabetes* 2003; 52:812–817.

[27] Hu FB, Meigs JB, Li TY, Rifai N, Manson JE. Inflammatory markers and risk of developing type 2 diabetes in women. *Diabetes* 2004;53:693-700.

[28] Herder C, Illig T, Rathmann W, Martin S, Haastert B, Müller-Scholze S, Holle R, Thorand B, Koenig W, Wichmann HE, Kolb H, for the KORA Study Group. Inflammation and type 2 diabetes: Results from KORA Augsburg. Gesundheitswesen 2005;67(Suppl. 1):S115-S121.

[29] Uysal KT,Wiesbrock SM, MarinoMW, Hotamisligil GS. Protection from obesity-induced insulin resistance in mice lacking TNF-alpha function. *Nature* 1997;389:610–614.

[30] Dong ZM, Gutierrez-Ramos JC, Coxon A, Mayadas TN, Wagner DD. A new class of obesity genes encodes leukocyte adhesion receptors. *Proc. Natl. Acad. Sci. USA* 1997;94:7526-7530.

[31] Schafer K, Fujisawa K, Konstantinides S, Loskutoff DJ. Disruption of the plasminogen activator inhibitor 1 gene reduces the adiposity and improves the metabolic profile of genetically obese and diabetic ob/ob mice. *FASEB J.* 2001;15:1840–1842.

[32] Perreault M, Marette A. Targeted disruption of inducible nitric oxide synthase protects against obesity-linked insulin resistance in muscle. *Nat. Med.* 2001;7:1138–1143.

[33] Wallenius V, Wallenius K, Ahren B, Rudling M, Carlsten H, Dickson SL, Ohlsson C, Jansson JO. Interleukin-6-deficient mice develop mature-onset obesity. *Nat. Med.* 2002;8:75–79.

[34] Ma LJ, Mao SL, Taylor KL, Guan Y, Zhang Y, Brown NJ, Swift LL, McGuinness OP, Wasserman DH, Vaughan DE, Fogo AB. Prevention of obesity and insulin resistance in mice lacking plasminogen activator inhibitor 1. *Diabetes* 2004;53:336–346.

[35] Rich SS, French LR, Sprafka JM, Clements JP, Goetz FC. HLA-associated susceptibility to type 2 (non-insulin-dependent) diabetes mellitus: the Wadena City Health Study. *Diabetologia* 1993;36:234–238.

[36] Tuomilehto-Wolf E, Tuomilehto J, Hitman GA, Nissinen A, Stengård J, Pekkanen J, Kivinen P, Kaarsalo E, Karvonen MJ. Genetic susceptibility to non-insulin dependent diabetes mellitus and glucose intolerance are located in HLA region. *BMJ* 1993;307:155–159.

[37] Ghabanbasani MZ, Spaepen M, Buyse I, Legius E, Decorte R, Bex M, Marynen P, Bouillon R, Cassiman JJ. Increased and decreased relative risk for non-insulin-dependent diabetes mellitus conferred by HLA class II and by CD4 alleles. *Clin. Genet* 1995;47:225–230.

[38] Metcalfe KA, Hitman GA, Pociot F, Bergholdt R, Tuomilehto-Wolf E, Tuomilehto J, Viswanathan M, Ramachandran A, Nerup J. An association between type 1 diabetes and the interleukin-1 receptor type 1 gene. The DiMe Study Group. Childhood Diabetes in Finland. *Hum. Immunol.* 1996;51:41-48.

[39] Fernandez-Real JM, Vendrell J, Ricart W, Broch M, Gutiérrez C, Casamitjana R, Oriola J, Richart C. Polymorphism of the tumor necrosis factor-alpha receptor 2 gene is associated with obesity, leptin levels, and insulin resistance in young subjects and diet-treated type 2 diabetic patients. *Diabetes Care* 2000;23:831–837.

[40] Perez-Luque E, Alaez C, Malacara JM, Garay ME, Fajardo ME, Nava LE, Gorodezky C. Protective effect of DRB1 locus against type 2 diabetes mellitus in Mexican Mestizos. *Hum. Immunol.* 2003;64:110–118.

[41] Wolford JK, Gruber JD, Ossowski VM, Vozarova B, Antonio Tataranni P, Bogardus C, Hanson RL. A C-reactive protein promoter polymorphism is associated with type 2 diabetes mellitus in Pima Indians. *Mol. Genet Metab.* 2003;78:136–144.

[42] Vozarova B, Fernández-Real JM, Knowler WC, Gallart L, Hanson RL, Gruber JD, Ricart W, Vendrell J, Richart C, Tataranni PA, Wolford JK. The interleukin-6 (-174) G/C promoter polymorphism is associated with type-2 diabetes mellitus in Native Americans and Caucasians. *Hum. Genet* 2003;112:409-413.

[43] Asano K, Ikegami H, Fujisawa T, Nishino M, Nojima K, Kawabata Y, Noso S, Hiromine Y, Fukai A, Ogihara T. Molecular scanning of interleukin-21 gene and genetic susceptibility to type 1 diabetes. *Hum. Immunol.* 2007;68:384-391.

[44] Qi L, Rifai N, Hu FB. Interleukin-6 receptor gene, plasma C-reactive protein, and diabetes risk in women. *Diabetes.* 2009;58:275-278.

[45] Herder C, Peltonen M, Koenig W, Kräft I, Müller-Scholze S, Martin S, Lakka T, Ilanne-Parikka P, Eriksson JG, Hämäläinen H, Keinänen-Kiukaanniemi S, Valle TT, Uusitupa M, Lindström J, Kolb H, Tuomilehto J. Systemic immune mediators and lifestyle changes in the prevention of type 2 diabetes: results from the Finnish Diabetes Prevention Study. *Diabetes* 2006;55:2340-2346.

[46] Freeman DJ, Norrie J, Naveed S, Neely DG, Cobbe SM, Ford I, Isles C, Lorimer AR, Macfarlane PW, McKillop JH, Packard CJ, Shepherd J, Gaw A. Pravastatin and the development of diabetes mellitus: evidence for a protective treatment effect in the West of Scotland Coronary Prevention Study. *Circulation* 2001;103: 357–362.

[47] Weitz-Schmidt G. Statins as anti-inflammatory agents. *Trends Pharmacol.* Sci 2002;23: 482–486.

[48] McFarlane SI, Muniyappa R, Francisco R, Stowers JR. Pleiotropic effects of statins: lipid reduction and beyond. *J. Clin. Endocrinol. Metab* 2002;87:1451–1458.

[49] Levin K, Hother-Nielsen O, Henriksen JE, Beck-Nielsen H. Effects of troglitazone in young firstdegree relatives of patients with type 2 diabetes. *Diabetes Care* 2004:27:148–154.

[50] Anderson DC Jr. Pharmacologic prevention or delay of type 2 diabetes mellitus. *Ann. Pharmacother* 2005;39:102–109.

[51] Ricote M, Li AC, Wilson TM, Kelly CJ, Glass CK. The peroxisome proliferator-activated receptor-γ is a negative regulator of macrophage activation. *Nature* 1998;391:79–82.

[52] Jiang C, Ting AT, Seed B. PPAR-γ agonists inhibit production of monocyte inflammatory cytokines. *Nature* 1998;391:82–85.

[53] Haffner SM, Greenberg AS, Weston WM, Chen H, Williams K, Freed MI. Effect of rosiglitazone treatment on non-traditional markers of cardiovascular disease in patients with type 2 diabetes mellitus. *Circulation* 2002;106:679–684.

[54] Pickup JC, Mattock MB, Chusney GD, Burt D. NIDDM as a disease of the innate immune system: association of acute phase reactants and interleukin-6 with metabolic syndrome X. *Diabetologia* 1997;40:1286–1292.

[55] Pickup JC, Crook MA. Is type II diabetes mellitus a disease of the innate immune system? *Diabetologia* 1998;41:1241–124.

[56] Pickup JC. Inflammation and activated innate immunity in the pathogenesis of type 2 diabetes. *Diabetes Care* 2004;27:813-823.

[57] King GL. The role of inflammatory cytokines in diabetes and its complications. *J. Periodontol.* 2008;79(Suppl. 8):1527-1534.

[58] Cameron NE, Cotter MA. Pro-inflammatory mechanisms in diabetic neuropathy: focus on the nuclear factor kappa B pathway. *Curr. Drug Targets* 2008;9:60-67.

[59] Skindric DS, Lisak RP. Role of neuropoietic cytokines in development and progression of diabetic polyneuropathy: from glucose metabolism to neurodegeneration. *Exp. Diabesity Res.* 2003;4:303-312.

[60] Satoh J, Yagihashi S, Toyota T. The possible role of tumor necrosis factor-alpha in diabetic polyneuropathy. *Exp. Diabesity Res* 2003;4:65-71.

[61] Joussen AM, Poulaki V, Le ML, Koizumi K, Esser C, Janicki H, Schraermeyer U, Kociok N, Fauser S, Kirchhof B, Kern TS, Adamis AP. A central role for inflammation in the pathogenesis of diabetic retinopathy. *FASEB J.* 2004;18:1450-1452.

[62] Kern TS. Contributions of inflammatory processes to the development of the early stages of diabetic retinopathy. *Exp. Diabetes Res.* 2007;2007:95103.

[63] Adamis AP, Berman AJ. Immunological mechanisms in the pathogenesis of diabetic retinopathy. *Semin. Immunopathol* 2008;30:65-84.

[64] Kowluru RA, Odenbach S. Role of interleukin-1beta in the pathogenesis of diabetic retinopathy. *Br. J. Ophthalmol.* 2004;88:1343-1347.

[65] Krady JK, Basu A, Allen CM, Xu Y, LaNoue KF, Gardner TW, Levison SW. Minocycline reduces proinflammatory cytokine expression, microglial activation, and caspase-3 activation in a rodent model of diabetic retinopathy. *Diabetes* 2005;54:1559-1565.

[66] Joussen AM, Poulaki V, Mitsiades N, Kirchhof B, Koizumi K, Döhmen S, Adamis AP. Nonsteroidal anti-inflammatory drugs prevent early diabetic retinopathy via TNF-α suppression. *FASEB J.* 2002;16:438-440.

[67] Funatsu H, Yamashita H, Noma H, Mimura T, Nakamura S, Sakata K, Hori S. Aqueous humor levels of cytokines are related to vitreous levels and progression of diabetic retinopathy in diabetic patients. *Grafes Arch. Clin Exp. Ophthalmol.* 2005;243:3-8.

[68] Hernández C, Segura RM, Fonollosa A, Carrasco E, Francisco G, Simo R. Interleukin-8, monocyte chemoattractant protein-1 and IL-10 in the vitreous fluid of patients with proliferative diabetic retinopathy. *Diabet Med.* 2005;22:719-722.

[69] Forbes JM, Fukami K, Cooper ME. Diabetic nephropathy: where hemodynamics meets metabolism. *Exp. Clin. Endocrinol Diabetes* 2007;115:69–84.

[70] Maric C. Vasoactive hormones and the diabetic kidney. *ScientificWorldJournal* 2008;8:470–485.

[71] Wolf G. New insights into the pathophysiology of diabetic nephropathy: from haemodynamics to molecular pathology. *Eur. J. Clin. Invest* 2004;34:785-796.

[72] Martini S, Eichinger F, Nair V, Kretzler M. Defining human diabetic nephropathy on the molecular level: integration of transcriptomic profiles with biological knowledge. *Rev. Endocr. Metab Disord.* 2008 Dec;9:267-274.

[73] Tuttle KR. Linking metabolism and immunology: Diabetic nephropathy is an inflammatory disease. *J. Am. Soc. Nephrol.* 2005;16:1537-1538.

[74] Galkina E, Ley K. Leukocyte recruitment and vascular injury in diabetic nephropathy. *J. Am. Soc. Nephrol.* 2006;17:368-377.

[75] Tesch GH. Role of macrophages in complications of type 2 diabetes. *Clin. Exp. Pharmacol. Physiol.* 2007;34:1016-1019.

[76] Shikata K, Makino H. Role of macrophages in the pathogenesis of diabetic nephropathy. *Contrib. Nephrol.* 2001;134:46-54.

[77] Bohle A, Wehrmann M, Bogenschutz O, Batz C, Muller CA, Muller GA. The pathogenesis of chronic renal failure in diabetic nephropathy. Investigation of 488 cases of diabetic glomerulosclerosis. *Pathol. Res. Pract* 1991;187:251–259.

[78] Furuta T, Saito T, Ootaka T, Soma J, Obara K, Abe K, Yoshinaga K. The role of macrophages in diabetic glomerulosclerosis. *Am. J. Kidney Dis*. 1993;21:480–485.

[79] Sassy-Prigent C, Heudes D, Mandet C, Belair MF, Michel O, Perdereau B, Bariety J, Bruneval P. Early glomerular macrophage recruitment in streptozotocin-induced diabetic rats. *Diabetes* 2000;49:466–475.

[80] Chow F, Ozols E, Nikolic-Paterson DJ, Atkins RC, Tesch GH. Macrophages in mouse type 2 diabetic nephropathy: Correlation with diabetic state and progressive renal injury. *Kidney Int* 2004;65:116–128.

[81] Bending JJ, Lobo-Yeo A, Vergani D, Viberti GC. Proteinuria and activated T-lymphocytes in diabetic nephropathy. *Diabetes* 1988;37:507–511.

[82] Moriya R, Manivel JC, Mauer M. Juxtaglomerular apparatus T-cell infiltration affects glomerular structure in type 1 diabetic patients. *Diabetologia* 2004;47: 82–88.

[83] Sugimoto H, Shikata K, Hirata K, Akiyama K, Matsuda M, Kushiro M, Shikata Y, Miyatake N, Miyasaka M, Makino H. Increased expression of intercellular adhesion molecule-1 (ICAM-1) in diabetic rat glomeruli: Glomerular hyperfiltration is a potential mechanism of ICAM-1 upregulation. *Diabetes* 1997;46:2075–2081.

[84] Matsui H, Suzuki M, Tsukuda R, Iida K, Miyasaka M, Ikeda H. Expression of ICAM-1 on glomeruli is associated with progression of diabetic nephropathy in a genetically obese diabetic rat, Wistar fatty. *Diabetes Res. Clin. Pract* 1996;32:1–9.

[85] Coimbra TM, Janssen U, Grone HJ, Ostendorf T, Kunter U, Schmidt H, Brabant G, Floege J: Early events leading to renal injury in obese Zucker (fatty) rats with type II diabetes. *Kidney Int* 2000;57:167–182.

[86] Chow FY, Nikolic-Paterson DJ, Ozols E, Atkins RC, Tesch GH: Intercellular adhesion molecule-1 deficiency is protective against nephropathy in type 2 diabetic db/db mice. *J. Am. Soc. Nephrol*. 2005;16:1711–1722.

[87] Imani F, Horii Y, Suthanthiran M, Skolnik EY, Makita Z, Sharma V, Sehajpal P, Vlassara H. Advanced glycosylation endproduct-specific receptors on human and rat T-lymphocytes mediate synthesis of interferon gamma: Role in tissue remodeling. *J. Exp. Med.* 1993;178:2165–2172.

[88] Fardon NJ, Wilkinson R, Thomas TH. Abnormalities in primary granule exocytosis in neutrophils from type I diabetic patients with nephropathy. *Clin. Sci.* (Lond) 2002;102:69-75.

[89] Takahashi T, Hato F, Yamane T, Inaba M, Okuno Y, Nishizawa Y, Kitagawa S. Increased spontaneous adherence of neutrophils from type 2 diabetic patients with overt proteinuria: Possible role of the progression of diabetic nephropathy. *Diabetes Care* 2000;23:417-418.

[90] Medzhitov R, Preston-Hurlburt P, Janeway CA Jr. A human homologue of the Drosophila Toll protein signals activation of adaptive immunity. *Nature* 1997;388:394–397.

[91] Abreu MT, Arditi M. Innate immunity and toll-like receptors: clinical implications of basic science research. *J. Pediatr.* 2004;144:421– 429.

[92] Akira S, Uematsu S, Takeuchi O. Pathogen recognition and innate immunity. *Cell* 124:783–801.

[93] Andreakos E, Foxwell B, Feldmann ML. Is targeting toll-like receptors and their signaling pathway a useful therapeutic approach to modulating cytokine-driven inflammation? *Immunol. Rev.* 2004;202:250–265.

[94] Akira S, Takeda K. Toll-like receptor signaling. *Nat. Rev. Immunol.* 2005;4:499-511.

[95] Kaisho T, Akira S. Toll-like receptor function and signaling. *J. Allergy Clin. Immunol.* 2006;117:979–987.

[96] Frantz S, Ertl G, Bauersachs J. Mechanisms of disease: Toll-like receptors in cardiovascular disease. *Nat. Clin. Pract Cardiovasc. Med.* 2007;4:444-454.

[97] Kanczkowski W, Ziegler CG, Zacharowski K, Bornstein SR. Toll-like receptors in endocrine disease and diabetes. *Neuroimmunomodulation* 2008;15:54-60.

[98] Anders HJ, Banas B, Schlöndorff D. Signaling Danger: Toll-Like Receptors and their Potential Roles in Kidney Diseases. *J. Am. Soc. Nephrol.* 2004;15; 854-867.

[99] Anders HJ, Schlöndorff D. Toll-like receptors: emerging concepts in kidney disease. *Curr. Opin. Nephrol. Hypertens* 2007;16:177-183.

[100] Pawar RD, Patole PS, Zecher D, Segerer S, Kretzler M, Schlöndorff D, Anders HJ. Toll-Like Receptor-7 Modulates Immune Complex Glomerulonephritis. *J. Am. Soc. Nephrol.* 2006;17:141-149.

[101] Goldstein DR, Tesar BM, Akira S, Lakkis FG. Critical role of the Toll-like receptor signal adaptor protein MyD88 in acute allograft rejection. *J. Clin. Invest* 2003;111:1571-1578.

[102] Tsuboi N, Yoshikai Y, Matsuo S, Kikuchi T, Iwami K, Nagai Y, Takeuchi O, Akira S, Matsuguchi T. Roles of toll-like receptors in C-C chemokine production by renal tubular epithelial cells. *J. Immunol.* 2002;169:2026–2033.

[103] Cines DB, Pollak ES, Buck CA, Loscalzo J, Zimmerman GA, McEver RP, Pober JS, Wick TM, Konkle BA, Schwarts BS, Marnathan ES, McCrae KR, Hug BA, Schmidt A-M, Stern DM. Endothelial cells in physiology and in the pathophysiology of vascular disorders. *Blood* 1998;91:3527–3561.

[104] Middleton J, Patterson AM, Gardner L, Schmutz C, Ashton BA. Leukocyte extravasation: chemokine transport and presentation by the endothelium. *Blood* 2002;100:3853–3860.

[105] Moser B, Loetscher P. Lymphocyte traffic control by chemokines. *Nat. Immunol* 2001;2:123–128.

[106] Worthylake RA, Burridge K. Leukocyte transendothelial migration: orchestrating the underlying molecular machinery. *Curr. Opin. Cell Biol.* 2001;13:569–577.
[107] Murdoch C, Finn A. Chemokine receptors and their role in inflammation and infectious diseases. *Blood* 2000;95:3032–3043.
[108] Gerard C, Rollins BJ. Chemokine and disease. *Nat. Immunol.* 2001;2:108–115.
[109] Proudfoot AEI. Chemokine receptors: multifaceted therapeutic targets. *Nat. Rev. Immunol.* 2002;2:106–115.
[110] Segerer S, Alpers CE. Chemokines and chemokine receptors in renal pathology. *Curr. Opin. Nephrol Hypertens* 2003;12:243-249.
[111] Ruster C, Wolf G. The role of chemokines and chemokine receptors in diabetic nephropathy. *Front Biosci.* 2008;13:944-955.
[112] Rovin BH, Doe N, Tan LC. Monocyte chemoattractant protein-1 levels in patients with glomerular disease. *Am. J. Kidney Dis.* 1996;27:640–646.
[113] Banba N, Nakamura T, Matsumura M, Kuroda H, Hattori Y, Kasai K. Possible relationship of monocyte chemoattractant protein-1 with diabetic nephropathy. *Kidney Int* 2000;58:684-690.
[114] Wada T, Furuichi K, Sakai N, Iwata Y, Yoshimoto K, Shimizu M, Takeda SI, Takasawa K, Yoshimura M, Kida H, Kobayashi KI, Mukaida N, Naito T, Matsushima K, Yokoyama H. Up-regulation of MCP-1 in tubulointerstitial lesions of human diabetic nephropathy. *Kidney Int* 2000;58:1492-1498.
[115] Chiarelli F, Cipollone F, Mohn A, Marini M, Iezzi A, Fazia M, Tumini S, De Cesare D, Pomilio M, Pierdomenico SD, Di Gioacchino M, Cuccurullo F, Mezzetti A. Circulating monocyte chemoattractant protein-1 and early development of nephropathy in type 1 diabetes. *Diabetes Care* 2002;25:1829-1834.
[116] Takebayashi K, Matsumoto S, Aso Y, Inukai T. Association between circulating monocyte chemoattractant protein-1 and urinary albumin excretion in nonobese Type 2 diabetic patients. *J. Diabetes Complications* 2006;20:98-104.
[117] Tashiro K, Koyanagi I, Saitoh A, Shimizu A, Shike T, Ishiguro C, Koizumi M, Funabiki K, Horikoshi S, Shirato I, Tomino I. Urinary levels of monocyte chemoattractant protein-1 (MCP-1) and interleukin-8 (IL-8), and renal injuries in patients with type 2 diabetic nephropathy. *J. Clin. Lab Anal.* 2002;16:1-4.
[118] Morii T, Fujita H, Narita T, Shimotomai T, Fujishima H, Yoshioka N, Imai H, Kakei M, Ito S. Association of monocyte chemoattractant protein-1 with renal tubular damage in diabetic nephropathy. *J. Diabetes Complications* 2003;17:11-15.
[119] Chow FY, Nikolic-Paterson DJ, Ozols E, Atkins RC, Rollin BJ, Tesch GH. Monocyte chemoattractant protein-1 promotes the development of diabetic renal injury in streptozotocin-treated mice. *Kidney Int* 2006;69:73-80.
[120] Chow FY, Nikolic-Paterson DJ, Ma FY, Ozols E, Rollins BJ, Tesch GH. Monocyte chemoattractant protein-1-induced tissue inflammation is critical for the development of renal injury but not type 2 diabetes in obese db/db mice. *Diabetologia* 2007;50:471-480.
[121] Tesch GH. MCP-1/CCL2: a new diagnostic marker and therapeutic target for progressive renal injury in diabetic nephropathy. *Am. J. Physiol. Renal Physiol.* 2008;294:F697-701.

[122] Kanamori H, Matsubara T, Mima A, Sumi E, Nagai K, Takahashi T, Abe H, Iehara N, Fukatsu A, Okamoto H, Kita T, Doi T, Arai H. Inhibition of MCP-1/CCR2 pathway ameliorates the development of diabetic nephropathy. *Biochem. Biophys. Res. Commun.* 2007;360:772-777.

[123] Amann R, Tinzmann R, Angelkort B. ACE inhibitors improve diabetic nephropathy through suppression of renal MCP-1. *Diabetes Care* 2003;26:2421-2425.

[124] Han SY, Kim CH, Kim HS, Jee YH, Song HK, Lee MH, Han KH, Kim HK, Kang YS, Han JY, Kim YS, Cha DR. Spironolactone prevents diabetic nephropathy through an anti-inflammatory mechanism in type 2 diabetic rats. *J. Am. Soc. Nephrol* 2006;17:1362–1372.

[125] Takebayashi K, Matsumoto S, Aso Y, Inukai T. Aldosterone blockade attenuates urinary monocyte chemoattractant protein-1 and oxidative stress in patients with type 2 diabetes complicated by diabetic nephropathy. *J. Clin. Endocrinol. Metab.* 2006;91:2214–2217.

[126] F. Bazan, K. B. Bacon, G. Hardiman, W. Wang, K. Soo, D. Rossi, D. R. Greaves, A. Zlotnik and T. J. Schall: A new class of membrane-bound chemokine with a CX3C motif. *Nature* 1997;385:640-644.

[127] Umehara H, Bloom ET, Okazaki T, Nagano Y, Yoshie O, Imai T. Fractalkine in vascular biology: from basic research to clinical disease. *Arterioscler Thromb. Vasc. Biol.* 2004;24:34-40.

[128] Cybulsky MI, Hegele RA. The fractalkine receptor CX3CR1 is a key mediator of atherogenesis. *J. Clin. Invest.* 2003;111:1118–1120.

[129] Robinson LA, Nataraj C, Thomas DW, Howell DN, Griffiths R, Bautch V, Patel DD, Feng L, Coffman TM. A role for fractalkine and its receptor (CX3CR1) in cardiac allograft rejection. *J. Immunol.* 2000;165:6067–6072.

[130] Chen S, Bacon KB, Li L, Garcia GE, Xia Y, Lo D, Thompson DA, Siani MA, Yamamoto T, Harrison JK, Feng L. In vivo inhibition of CC and CX3C chemokine-induced leukocyte infiltration and attenuation of glomerulonephritis in Wistar-Kyoto (WKY) rats by vMIP-II. *J. Exp. Med.* 1998;188:193–198.

[131] Furuichi K, Wada T, Iwata Y, Sakai N, Yoshimoto K, Shimizu M, Kobayashi K, Takasawa K, Kida H, Takeda S, Matsushima K, Yokoyama H. Upregulation of fractalkine in human crescentic glomerulonephritis. *Nephron* 2000;87:314–320.

[132] Ito Y, Kawachi H, Morioka Y, Nakatsue T, koike H, Ikezuni Y, Oyanagi A, Natori Y, Natori Y, Nakamura T, Gejyo F, Shimizu F. Fractalkine expression and the recruitment of CX3CR1+ cells in the prolonged mesangial proliferative glomerulonephritis. *Kidney Int* 2002;61:2044–2057.

[133] Segerer S, Hughes E, Hudkins KL, Mack M, Goodpaster T, Alpers CE. Expression of the fractalkine receptor (CX3CR1) in human kidney disease. *Kidney Int* 2002;62:488–495.

[134] Cockwell P, Chakravorty SJ, Girdlestone J, Savage COS. Fractalkine expression in human renal inflammation. *J. Pathol.* 2002;196:85–90.

[135] Ruth JH, Volin MV, Haines GK III, Woodruff DC, Katschke KJ Jr, Woods JM, Park CC, Morel JCM, Koch AE. Fractalkine, a novel chemokine in rheumatoid arthritis and in rat adjuvant-induced arthritis. *Arthritis Rheum* 2001;44:1568–1581.

[136] Volin MV, Woods JM, Amin MA, Connors MA, Harlow LA, Koch AE. Fractalkine: a novel angiogenic chemokine in rheumatoid arthritis. *Am. J. Pathol.* 2001;159:1521–1530.

[137] Raychaudhuri SP, Jiang W-Y, Farber EM. Cellular localization of fractalkine at sites of inflammation: antigen-presenting cells in psoriasis express high levels of fractalkine. *Br. J. Dermatol.* 2001;144:1105–1113.

[138] Balabanian K, Foussat A, Dormuller P, Durand-Gasselin I, Capel F, Bouchet-Delbos L, Portier A, Marfaing-Koka A, Krzysiek R, Rimaniol A-C, Simonneau G, Emilie D, Humbert M. CX3C chemokine fractalkine in pulmonary arterial hypertension. *Am. J. Respir Crit. Care Med.* 2002;165:1419–1425.

[139] Efsen E, Grappone C, DeFranco RMS, Milani S, Romanelli RG, Bonacchi A, Caligiuri A, Failli P, Annunziato F, Paglial G, Pinzani M, Laffi G, Gentilini P, Marra F. Up-regulated expression of fractalkine and its receptor CX3CR1 during liver injury in humans. *J. Hepatol.* 2002;37:39–47.

[140] Cardozo AK, Proost P, Gysemans C, Chen M-C, Mathieu C, Eizirik DL. IL-1β and IFN-γ induce the expression of diverse chemokines and IL-15 in human and rat pancreatic islet cells, and in islets from pre-diabetic NOD mice. *Diabetologia* 2003;46:255–266.

[141] Kikuchi Y, Ikee R, Hemmi N, Hyodo N, Saigusa T, Namikoshi T, Yamada M, Suzuki S, Miura S. Fractalkine and its receptor, CX3CR1, upregulation in streptozotocin-induced diabetic kidneys. *Nephron. Exp. Nephrol.* 2004;97:e17-25.

[142] Schall TJ Jongstra J, Dyer BJ, Jorgensen J, Clayberger C, Davis MM, Krensky AM. A human T cell-specific molecule is a member of a new gene family. *J. Immunol.* 1988;141:1018–1025.

[143] 143.Wolf G, Aberle S, Thaiss F, Nelson PJ, Krensky AM, Neilson EG, Stahl RA. TNF alpha induces expression of the chemoattractant cytokine RANTES in cultured mouse mesangial cells. *Kidney Int* 1993;44:795-804.

[144] 144.Heeger P, Wolf G, Meyers C, Sun MJ, O'Farrell MC, Krensky AM, Neilson EG. Isolation and characterization of cDNA from renal tubular epithelium encoding murine Rantes. *Kidney Int* 1992;41:220-225.

[145] 145.Satriano A, Banas B, Luckow B, Nelson P, Schlondorff D. Regulation of RANTES and ICAM-1 expression in murine mesangial cells. *J. Am. Soc. Nephrol.* 1997;8:596-603.

[146] Pattison J, Nelson PJ, Huie P, von Leuttichau I, Farshid G, Sibley RK, Krensky AM. RANTES chemokine expression in cell-mediated transplant rejection of the kidney. *Lancet* 1994;343:209–211.

[147] Herder C, Haastert B, Müller-Scholze S, Koenig W, Thorand B, Holle R, Wichmann HE, Scherbaum WA, Martin S, Kolb H. Association of systemic chemokine concentrations with impaired glucose tolerance and type 2 diabetes: results from the Cooperative Health Research in the Region of Augsburg Survey S4 (KORA S4). *Diabetes* 2005;54(Suppl 2):S11-S17.

[148] Herder C, Peltonen M, Koenig W, Kräft I, Müller-Scholze S, Martin S, Lakka T, Ilanne-Parikka P, Eriksson JG, Hämäläinen H, Keinänen-Kiukaanniemi S, Valle TT, Uusitupa M, Lindström J, Kolb H, Tuomilehto J. Systemic immune mediators and

lifestyle changes in the prevention of type 2 diabetes: results from the Finnish Diabetes Prevention Study. *Diabetes* 2006;55:2340-2346.

[149] Mezzano S, Aros C, Droguett A, Burgos ME, Ardiles L, Flores C, Schneider H, Ruiz-Ortega M, Egido J. NF-kappaB activation and overexpression of regulated genes in human diabetic nephropathy. *Nephrol Dial Transplant* 2004;19:2505-2512.

[150] Segerer S, MacK M, Regele H, Kerjaschki D, Schlondorff D. Expression of the C-C chemokine receptor 5 in human kidney diseases. *Kidney Int* 1999;56:52-64.

[151] Furuichi K, Wada T, Sakai N, Iwata Y, Yoshimoto K, Shimizu M, Kobayashi K, Takasawa K, Kida H, Takeda SI, Mukaida N, Matsushima K, Yokoyama H. Distinct expression of CCR1 and CCR5 in glomerular and interstitial lesions of human glomerular diseases. *Am. J. Nephrol*. 2000;20:291-299.

[152] Albelda SM, Smith CW, Ward PA. Adhesion molecules and inflammatory injury. *FASEB J.* 1994;8:504-512.

[153] Yang L, Froio RM, Sciuto TE, Dvorak AM, Alon R, Luscinskas FW. ICAM-1 regulates neutrophil adhesion and transcellular migration of TNF-alpha-activated vascular endothelium under flow. *Blood* 2005;106:584–592.

[154] Okada S, Shikata K, Matsuda M, Ogawa D, Usui H, Kido Y, Nagase R, Wada J, Shikata Y, Makino H. Intercellular adhesion molecule-1 deficient mice are resistant against renal injury after induction of diabetes. *Diabetes* 2003;52:2586–2593.

[155] Matsui H, Suzuki M, Tsukuda R, Iida K, Miyasaka M, Ikeda H. Expression of ICAM-1 on glomeruli is associated with rogression of diabetic nephropathy in a genetically obese diabetic rat, Wistar fatty. *Diabetes Res. Clin. Pract*. 1996;32:1–9.

[156] Coimbra TM, Janssen U, Grone HJ, Ostendorf T, Kunter U, Schmidt H, Brabant G, Floege J. Early events leading to renal injury in obese Zucker (fatty) rats with type II diabetes. *Kidney Int* 2000; 57:167–182.

[157] Clausen P, Jacobsen P, Rossing K, Jensen JS, Parving HH, Feldt-Rasmussen B. Plasma concentrations of VCAM-1 and ICAM-1 are elevated in patients with type1 diabetes mellitus with microalbuminuria and overt nephropathy. *Diabet Med* 2000;17: 644–649.

[158] Guler S, Cakir B, Demirbas B, Yönem A, Odabasi E, Onde U, Aykut O, Gürsoy G. Plasma soluble intercellular adhesion molecules 1 levels are increased in type 2 diabetic patients with nephropathy. *Horm. Res*. 2002;58:67–70.

[159] Ina K, Kitamura H, Okeda T, Nagai K, Liu ZY, Matsuda M, Fujikura Y. Vascular cell adhesion molecule-1 expression in the renal interstitium of diabetic KKAy mice. *Diabetes Res. Clin. Pract* 1999;44:1-8.

[160] Lim SC, Caballero AE, Smakowski P, LoGerfo FW, Horton ES, Veves A. Soluble intercellular adhesion molecule, vascular cell adhesion molecule, and impaired microvascular reactivity are early markers of vasculopathy in type 2 diabetic individuals without microalbuminuria. *Diabetes Care* 1999;22: 1865–1870.

[161] Schmidt AM, Crandall J, Hori O, Cao R, Lakatta E. Elevated plasma levels of vascular cell adhesion molecule-1 (VCAM-1) in diabetic patients with microalbuminuria: a marker of vascular dysfunction and progressive vascular disease. *Br. J. Haematol* 1996;92:747–750.

[162] Stehouwer CD, Gall MA, Twisk JW, Knudsen E, Emeis JJ, Parving HH. Increased urinary albumin excretion, endothelial dysfunction, and chronic low-grade

inflammation in type 2 diabetes: progressive, interrelated, and independently associated with risk of death. *Diabetes* 2002;51:1157–1165.

[163] Coen D, Stehouwer A, Gall MA, Twisk JWR, Knudsen E, Emeis JJ, Parving HH. Increased Urinary Albumin Excretion, Endothelial Dysfunction, and Chronic Low-Grade Inflammation in Type 2 Diabetes. *Diabetes* 2002;51:1157-1165.

[164] Ryan US, Worthington RE. Cell-cell contact mechanisms. *Curr. Opin. Immunol* 1992;4:33–37.

[165] Hirata K, Shikata K, Matsuda M, Akiyama K, Sugimoto H, Kushiro M, Makino H. Increased expression of selectins in kidneys of patients with diabetic nephropathy. *Diabetologia* 1998;41:185-192.

[166] Narumi S, Onozato ML, Tojo A, Sakamoto S, Tamatani T. Tissue-specific induction of E-selectin in glomeruli is augmented following diabetes mellitus. *Nephron* 2001;89:161-171.

[167] Soedamah-Muthu SS, Chaturvedi N, Schalkwijk CG, Stehouwer CD, Ebeling P, Fuller JH. Soluble vascular cell adhesion molecule-1 and soluble E-selectin are associated with micro- and macrovascular complications in type 1 diabetic patients. *J. Diabet. Complications* 2006;20:188–195.

[168] Lopes-Virella MF, Carter RE, Gilbert GE, Klein RL, Jaffa M, Jenkins AJ, Lyons TJ, Garvey WT, Virella G; Diabetes Control and Complications Trial/Epidemiology of Diabetes Intervention and Complications Cohort Study Group. Risk factors related to inflammation and endothelial dysfunction in the DCCT/EDIC cohort and their relationship with nephropathy and macrovascular complications. *Diabetes Care* 2008;31:2006-2012.

[169] Welsch T, Endlich N, Kriz W, Endlich K. CD2AP and p130Cas localize to different F-actin structures in podocytes. *Am. J. Physiol. Renal. Physiol.* 2001;281: F769-777.

[170] Kigawa A, Wakui H, Maki N, Okuyama S, Masai R, Ohtani H, Komatsuda A, Suzuki D, Toyoda M, Kobayashi R, Sawada K. Interaction of the spectrin-like repeats of alpha-actinin-4 with humanin peptide. *Clin. Exp. Nephrol.* 2004;8:331-338.

[171] Dandapani SV, Sugimoto H, Matthews BD, Kolb RJ, Sinha S, Gerszten RE, Zhou J, Ingber DE, Kalluri R, Pollak MR. Alpha-actinin-4 is required for normal podocyte adhesion. *J. Biol. Chem.* 2007;282:467-477.

[172] Kimura M, Toyoda M, Kato M, Kobayashi K, Abe M, Kobayashi T, Miyauchi M, Yamamoto N, Umezono T, Suzuki D. Expression of alpha-actinin-4 in human diabetic nephropathy. *Intern Med.* 2008;47:1099-106.

[173] Balwilk FR, Burke F. The cytokine network. *Immunol Today* 1989;10:299-304.

[174] Coppack SW. Pro-inflammatory cytokines and adipose tissue. *Proc. Nutr. Soc.* 2001;60:349–356.

[175] AldhahiW, Hamdy O. Adipokines, inflammation, and the endothelium in diabetes. *Curr. Diab. Rep.* 2003;3:293–298.

[176] Hasegawa G, Nakano K, Sawada M, Uno K, Shibayama Y, Ienaga K, Kondo M. Possible role of tumor necrosis factor and interleukin-1 in the development of diabetic nephropathy. *Kidney Int* 1991;40:1007-1012.

[177] Hasegawa G, Nakano K, Kondo M. Role of TNF and IL-1 in the development of diabetic nephropathy. *Nefrologia* 1995;15:1-4.

[178] Nakamura T, Fukui M, Ebihara I, Osada S, Nagaoka I, Tomino Y, Koide H. mRNA expression of growth factors in glomeruli from diabetic rats. *Diabetes* 1993;42:450-456.

[179] Sugimoto H, Shikata K, Wada J, Horiuchi S, Makino H. Advanced glycation end products-cytokine-nitric oxide sequence pathway in the development of diabetic nephropathy: aminoguanidine ameliorates the overexpression of tumour necrosis factor-alpha and inducible oxide synthase in diabetic rat glomerli. *Diabetologia* 1999;42:878-886.

[180] Sassy-Prigent C, Heudes D, Jouquey S, Auberval D, Belair MF, Michel O, Hamon G, Bariety J, Bruneval P. Early glomerular macrophage recruitment in streptozotocin-induced diabetic rats. *Diabetes* 2000;49:466-475.

[181] Navarro JF, Milena FJ, Mora C, León C, García J. Renal pro-inflammatory cytokine gene expression in diabetic nephropathy: Effect of angiotensin-converting enzyme inhibition and pentoxifylline administration. *Am. J. Nephrol.* 2006;26:562-570.

[182] Brady HR. Leukocyte adhesion molecules and kidney diseases. *Kidney Int* 1994;45:1285-1300.

[183] Park CW, Kim JH, Lee JH, Kim YS, Ahn HJ, Shin YS, Kim SY, Choi EJ, Chang YS, Bang BK. High glucose-induced intercellular adhesion molecule-1 (ICAM-1) expression through an osmotic effect in rat mesangial cells is PKC-NFkapa B-dependent. *Diabetologia* 2000;43:1544-1553.

[184] Pfeilschifter J, Pignat W, Vosbeck K, Märki F. Interleukin 1 and tumor necrosis factor synergistically stimulate prostaglandin synthesis and phospholipase A2 release from rat renal mesangial cells. *Biochem. Biophys. Res. Commun.* 1989;159:385-394.

[185] Pfeilschifter J, Mühl H. Interleukin-1 and tumor necrosis factor potentiate angiotensin II- and calcium ionophore-stimulated prostaglandin E2 synthesis in rat renal mesangial cells. *Biochem. Biophys. Res. Commun.* 1990;169:585-595.

[186] Royall JA, Berkow RL, Beckman JS, Cunningham MK, Matalon S, Freeman BA. Tumor necrosis factor and interleukin 1 increase vascular endothelial permeability. *Am. J. Physiol.* 1989;257:L339-L410.

[187] Jones S, Jones S, Phillips AO. Regulation of renal proximal tubular epithelial cell hyaluronan generation: implications for diabetic nephropathy. *Kidney Int* 2001;59:1739-1749.

[188] Mahadevan P, Larkins RG, Fraser JR, Fosang AJ, Dunlop ME. Increased hyaluronan production in the glomeruli from diabetic rats: Link between glucose induced prostaglandin production and reduced sulphated proteoglycans. *Diabetologia* 1995;38:298–305.

[189] Sekizuka K, Tomino Y, Sei C, Kurusu A, Tashiro K, Yamaguchi Y, Kodera S, Hishiki T, Shirato I, Koide H. Detection of serum IL-6 in patients with diabetic nephropathy. *Nephron* 1994;68:284-285.

[190] Suzuki D, Miyazaki M, Naka R, Koji T, Yagame M, Endoh M, Sakai H. In situ hybridization of interleukin 6 in diabetic nephropathy. *Diabetes* 1995;44:1233-1238.

[191] Nosadini R, Velussi, M, Brocco E, Bruseghin M, Abaterusso C, Saller A, Dalla Vestra M, Carraro A, Bortoloso E, Sambataro M, Barzon I, Frigato F, Muollo B, Chiesura-Corona M, Pacini G, Baggio B, Piarulli F, Sfriso A, Fioretto P. Course of renal function

in type 2 diabetic patients with abnormalities of albumin excretion rate. *Diabetes* 2000;49:476-484.

[192] Dalla Vestra M, Mussap M, Gallina P, Brueghin M, Cernigoi AM, Saller A, Plebani M, Fioretto P. Acute-phase markers of inflammation and glomerular structure in patients with type 2 diabetes. *J. Am. Soc. Nephrol.* 2005;16(Suppl 1):S78-S82.

[193] Thomson SC, Deng A, Bao D, Satriano J, Blantz RC, Vallon V. Ornithine decarboxylase, kidney size, and the tubular hypothesis of glomerular hyperfiltration in experimental diabetes. *J. Clin. Invest* 2001;107:217-224.

[194] Okamura H, Tsutsui H, Komatsu T, Yutsudo M, Hakura A, Tanimoto T, Torigoe K, Okura T, Nukada Y, Hattori K, Akita K, Namba M, Tanabe F, Konishi K, Fukuda S, Kurimoto M. Cloning a new cytokine that induces IFN-production by T cells. *Nature* 1995;378:88-91.

[195] Dai SM, Matsuno H, Nakamura H, Nishioka K, Yudoh K. Interleukin-18 enhances monocyte tumor necrosis factor alpha and interleukin-1 beta production induced by directo contact with T lymphocytes: implications in rheumatoid arthritis. *Arthritis Rheum.* 2004;50:432-443.

[196] Marino E, Cardier JE. Differential effects of IL-18 on endothelial cell apoptosis mediated by TNF-alpha and Fas (CD59). *Cytokine* 2003;22:142-148.

[197] Stuyt RJ, Netea MG, Geijtenbeek TB, Kullberg BJ, Dinarello CA, van der Meer JW. Selective regulation of intercellular adhesion molecule-1 expression by interleukin-18 and interleukin-12 on human monocytes. *Immunology* 2003;110:329-334.

[198] Fantuzzi G, Reed DA, Dinarello CA. IL-12-induced IFN-gamma is dependent of caspase-1 processing of the IL-18 precursor. *J. Clin. Invest* 1999;104:761-767.

[199] Melnikov VY, Ecder T, Fantuzzi G, Siegmund B, Lucia MS, Dinarello CA, Schrier RW, Edelstein CL. Impaired IL-18 processing protects caspase-1-deficient mice from ischemic acute renal failure. *J. Clin. Invest* 2001;107:1145-1152.

[200] Melnikov VY, Faubel S, Siegmund B, Lucia MS, Ljubanovic D, Edelstein CL. Neutrophil-independent mechanisms of caspase-1 and IL-18 mediated ischemic acute tubular necrosis in mice. *J. Clin. Invest* 2002;110:1083-1091.

[201] Moriwaki Y, Yamamoto T, Shibutani Y, Aoki E, Tsutsumi Z, Takahashi S, Okamura H, Koga M, Fukuchi M, Hada T. Elevated levels of interleukin-18 and tumor necrosis factor-α in serum of patients with type 2 diabetes mellitus: relationship with diabetic nephropathy. *Metabolism* 2003;52:605-608.

[202] Nakamura A, Shikata K, Hiramatsu M, Nakatou T, Kitamura T, Wada J, Itoshima T, Makino H. Serum interleukin-18 levels are associated with nephropathy and atherosclerosis in Japanese patients with type 2 diabetes. *Diabetes Care* 2005;28:2890-2895.

[203] Wong CK, Ho AWY, Tong PCY, Yeung CY, Kong APS, Lun SWM, Chan JCN, Lam CWK. Aberrant activation profile of cytokines and mitogen-activated protein kinases in type 2 diabetic patients with nephropathy. *Clin. Exp. Immunol.* 2007;149:123-131.

[204] Araki S, Haneda M, Koya D. Predictive impact of elevated serum level of IL-18 for early renal dysfunction in type 2 diabetes: an observational follow-up study. *Diabetologia* 2007;50:867-873.

[205] Wang X, Feuerstein GZ, Xu L, Wang H, Schumacher WA, Ogletree ML, Taub R, Duan JJ, Decicco CP, Liu RQ. Inhibition of tumor necrosis factor-alpha-converting enzyme by a selective antagonist protects brain from focal ischemic injury in rats. *Mol. Pharamcol.* 2004;65:890-896.

[206] Navarro J, Milena F, Mora C, Leon C, Claverie F, Flores C, Garcia J. Tumor necrosis factor-α gene expression in diabetic nephropathy: Relatioship with urinary albumin excretion and effect of angiotensin-converting enzyme inhibition. *Kidney Int* 2005;68(Suppl 99):S98-S102.

[207] Dipetrillo K, Coutermarsh B, Gesek FA. Urinary tumor necrosis factor contributes to sodium retention and renal hypertrophy during diabetes. *Am. J. Physiol. Renal. Physiol.* 2003;284:F113-121.

[208] Dipetrillo K, Gesek FA. Pentoxifylline ameliorates renal tumor necrosis factor expression, sodium retention, and renal hypertrophy in diabetic rats. *Am. J. Nephrol.* 2004;24:352-359.

[209] Bertani T, Abbate M, Zoja C, Corna D, Perico N, Ghezzi P, Remuzzi G. Tumor necrosis factor induces glomerular damage in rabbit. *Am. J. Pathol.* 1989;134:419–430.

[210] Baud L, Ardaillou R. Tumor necrosis factor in renal injury. *Miner Electrolyte Metab* 1995;21:336–341.

[211] Schreiner GF, Kohan DE. Regulation of renal transport processes and hemodynamics by macrophages and lymphocytes. *Am. J. Physiol.* 1990;258:F761-767.

[212] Kalantarinia K, Awas AS, Siragy HM. Urinary and renal interstitial concentrations of TNF-α increase prior to the rise in albuminuria in diabetic rats. *Kidney Int* 2003;64:1208-1213.

[213] Ortiz A, Bustos C, Alonso J, Alcázar R, López-Armada MJ, Plaza JJ, González E, Egido J. Involvement of tumor necrosis factor-alpha in the pathogenesis of experimental, and human glomerulonephritis. *Adv. Nephrol. Necker. Hosp.* 1995;24:53-77.

[214] Laster SM, Wood JG, Gooding LR. Tumor necrosis factor can induce both apoptotic and necrotic forms of cell lysis. *J. Immunol.* 1988:141:2629-2634.

[215] Boyle JJ, Weissberg PL, Bennett MR. Tumor necrosis factor-alpha promotes macrophage-induced vascular smooth muscle cell apoptosis by direct and autocrine mechanisms. *Arterioscler. Thromb. Vasc. Biol.* 2003;23:1553–1558.

[216] Baud L, Pérez J, Friedlander G, Ardaillou R. Tumor necrosis factor stimulates prostaglandin production and cyclic AMP levels in rat cultured mesangial cells. *FEBS Lett* 1998;239:50-54.

[217] Wojciak-Stothard B, Entwistle A, Garg R, and Ridley AJ. Regulation of TNF-alpha-induced reorganization of the actin cytoskeleton and cell-cell junctions by Rho, Rac, and Cdc42 in human endothelial cells. *J. Cell Physiol.* 1998;176:150–165.

[218] Raedke HH, Meier B, Topley N, Fluge J, Habermehl GG, Resch K. Interleukin 1-α and tumor necrosis factor-α induce oxygen radical production in mesangial cells. *Kidney Int* 1990;37:767-775.

[219] Koike N, Takamura T, Kaneko S. Induction of reactive oxygen species from isolated rat glomerli by protein kinase C activation and TNF-α stimulation, and effects of a phosphodiesterase inhibitor. *Life Sci.* 2007;80:1721-1728.

[220] MaCarthy E, Sharma R, Sharma M, Li JZ, Ge XL, Dileepan KN, Savin VJ. TNF-α increases albumin permeability of isolated rat glomeruli through the generation of superoxide. *J. Am. Soc. Nephrol.* 1998;9:433-438.
[221] Navarro JF, Mora C, Macía M, García J. Inflammatory parameters are independently associated with urinary albumin excretion in type 2 diabetes mellitus. *Am. J. Kidney Dis.* 2003;42:53-61.
[222] Navarro JF, Mora C, Muros M, García J. Urinary tumor necrosis factor-α is independently associated with clinical markers of renal injury in diabetic patients. *Nephrol. Dial Transplant* 2006;21:3428-3434.

In: Nephrology – Dialysis - Transplantation
Editors: Endre Kruger and Kelemen Hahn

ISBN 978-1-60741-736-1
© 2009 Nova Science Publishers, Inc.

Chapter II

Indexing Glomerular Filtration Rate for Body Surface Area: Myth and Reality

Pierre Delanaye[1], Christophe Mariat[2], Etienne Cavalier[3] and Jean-Marie Krzesinski[1]

[1]University of Liège
Department of Nephrology, Dialysis, Hypertension, Transplantation CHU Sart Tilman, Liège, Belgium
[2]University of Saint-Etienne
Department of Nephrology, Dialysis, Hypertension, Transplantation Hopital Nord, Saint-Etienne, France
[3]University of Liège
Department of Clinical Chemistry
CHU Sart Tilman, Liège, Belgium

Abstract

Indexing glomerular filtration rate (GFR) for body surface area (BSA) is often realized without arising any questions. However, physiological basis for such an indexation are very poor. Indeed, indexing GFR for BSA to avoid variation due to differences in body size necessarily implies that GFR is a linear function of BSA and that the intercept of this linear function is zero. Moreover, when GFR is indexed for BSA, the relation indexed GFR-BSA must completely disappear. These physiological prerequisites are not found for BSA indexation. We will review the history of this indexation and will underline errors and defaults. Different equations to estimate BSA exist and will be discussed. The choice of "1.73 m^2" will be also criticized. Moreover, indexing GFR for BSA has little impact on GFR results in "normal" body size population. Nevertheless, this indexation will have strong consequences in anorexia and in obese patients. These consequences will be illustrated by our original data. We will discuss possible alternatives proposed to substitute for BSA indexation.

Introduction

In this chapter, we will discuss an important but under-recognized topic in Nephrology. Indeed, indexing glomerular filtration rate (GFR) for body surface area (BSA) is often realized from force of habit, because everyone does it and without arising any questions…Relatively few literature on this topic has been published in the last decades and most of articles on this topic disown this indexation [1]. Regarding guidelines on estimating and measuring GFR, only the Australian ones deeply discuss this topic [2]. Indeed, indexing GFR is not free from criticisms and may be misleading, especially in some specific populations.

Why Indexing GFR for BSA? Good and Bad Reasons

There are only two good reasons for indexing GFR (or any other physiological data) by an anthropometrical measure (like BSA). The first and most important reason is to permit comparison of GFR measurements between subjects with different body size. Intuitively, one can't expect the same meaning from an absolute (i.e. non-indexed) GFR value obtained in Stan Laurel or Oliver Hardy [1,3,4].

The second reason is the establishment of "normal" reference value for GFR. It seems suitable that such references are common to all subjects from lean to obese and from babies to elderly people, but it is not free from criticisms (at least this reason is not sufficient) as we will further show [1,3]. If good reasons do exist for using indexed GFR, unfortunately, the bad reasons are often advanced (explicitly or not) in the literature. Indexing GFR for BSA is so accepted in the scientific community that its use is sometimes justified by non scientific arguments. One of such arguments used for justifying BSA indexing is that using it decreases dispersion of data. For example, use of indexing BSA in children makes the GFR data comparable to adults' data. As we will see in the mathematical paragraph, this argument is not sufficient and not supported by any scientific data [5,6]. Other arguments used in favour of indexing are still more distressing and absolutely not scientific. Indeed, most of authors use BSA indexing as a rule, without raising any questions and only because everybody uses it and also because it is so easy to use [6-9]. The fact that everybody uses BSA indexation would make the data from different studies comparable, as well. In this view, the use of BSA indexing is automatic, sometimes unconsciously. We reproduce here what Kronmal wrote in 1983 [9]: "Everyone else uses this ratio. If we don't, we won't be able to compare our results with those of others. Although this argument sounds like what one hears from a teenage to justify particularly noxious behaviour, it is equally difficult to counter in this context. The reviewers of the investigator's paper may have already published articles using this ratio and will sometimes insist that this is the only correct way to present the data. Thus the burden falls on the investigator and the statistician to explain why the presentation of the results without the ratio is preferable". From our own experience, we can state that such an affirmation is unfortunately still valid in 2009.

Indexing GFR for BSA: The Genesis

The founder article regarding indexation of GFR for BSA has been published in 1928 by McIntosh [10]. This author was also the first to use the factor 1.73m² for that indexation. As we will see further, it is important to underline that McIntosh used ideal weight (not measured) for estimating BSA. In this article, the author compared renal function (reflected by urea clearance) in 18 adults and 8 children (from 2 to 12 years old). Indexing GFR for BSA gave comparable urea clearance results between children and adults [10]. These data were confirmed in 1931 by Holten who studied 90 children and adolescents using creatinine clearance [11]. Once again, decreasing the dispersion of the data is not a strong argument for BSA indexing [5]. McIntosh had built his indexation theory with experience from earlier American physiological studies [10]. In 1923, Taylor described an "approximately" (the scientific vocabulary at the beginning of the 20th century is sometime surprising!) direct correlation between urea excretion (thought to reflect renal function at this time) and the weight of the kidney in 23 rabbits [12]. This author also described a better correlation between kidney weight and BSA than between kidney weight and animal's weight. Such a conclusion had also been given by Stewart on a limited number of dogs [13]. We have re-calculated correlation with data given by Taylor in his original article and noted that the correlation between BSA and kidney weight was not different from that between kidney weight and weight. In 1932, MacKay illustrated a direct correlation between BSA and kidney weight and between BSA and urea excretion in humans [14]. From these observations, McIntosh concluded that BSA was strongly correlated to renal function [10]. However, this conclusion may be viewed as too optimistic as BSA had not been directly compared to GFR (without talking about the limitation of using urea clearance as a GFR marker). Holten described a correlation between creatinine clearance and BSA but he thought that this relationship was not direct but linked to the common relation to basal metabolic rate (BMR). He based this hypothesis on studies showing that thyroidectomy decreased kidney weight on one hand and that giving thyroid hormones increased protein metabolism and kidney weight (see below)[11].

Whatever shortens used (kidney function = urea excretion = kidney weight = BSA) in studies from which McIntosh based his BSA indexing theory, this theory received great success [10]. Once again, the decreased dispersion of the data was a "proof" of the performance of the BSA indexing. Nevertheless, this argument may lead to some curiosities. So, indexing GFR for BSA makes GFR values comparable between adults and children or infants, at least of one or two years old. Indexed GFRs before one year are classically lower and several authors argue that it is linked to the time of maturation for the kidneys [7,15-19]. This concept of kidney maturation is based on GFR measurements although histological studies on healthy babies are, of course, lacking [17]. Nevertheless, the way the GFR is indexed in babies (for BSA or extracellular volume, BMR or height…all these variables well decreasing the dispersion of the data!) will influence the time of the maturation. This has been illustrated by Rubin in 1949: GFR values in children are similar to adults' values at 2 years if GFR is indexed for BSA, at 5 months if indexed for kidney weight, before 6 months if body weight is used and after several years if BMR or height is used for indexation. Rubin finally favoured for indexation with BSA because "it is the most commonly used in the literature" (disappointing argument!!)[7]. The argument of "decreasing dispersion of data" is thus questionable but can also cynically be used against the indexation. Indeed, indexing GFR induces differences in GFR normal values between men and women (logically as men are heavier) that will fully disappear if absolute GFR is used [6].

Now it appears to us fundamental to underline the mathematical prerequisites for choosing the indexation of a physiological data.

Indexing GFR for BSA: Physiological and Mathematical Points of View

The physiological and mathematical prerequisites for the choice of GFR indexation are relatively easy to understand. If BSA is considered as a candidate for indexing GFR, two conditions must be present. Firstly, the relationship between GFR and BSA must be strong and linear (slope not different from 1). Straight line must pass through the 0 point (no intercept). The second prerequisite is also logical. The relationship between GFR and BSA must totally disappear when GFR is indexed for BSA (Figure 1)[4-6,9,20-22]. Several authors had well shown that these two conditions were poorly met regarding BSA and GFR [4,6,21-24]. For example, Dooley described a very poor correlation (r=0.22) between GFR (measured by isotopic reference method) and BSA in his population (n=122)[22]. Turner confirmed these results especially insisting on the fact that the slope of regression of the indexed GFR on BSA was actually not zero [6].

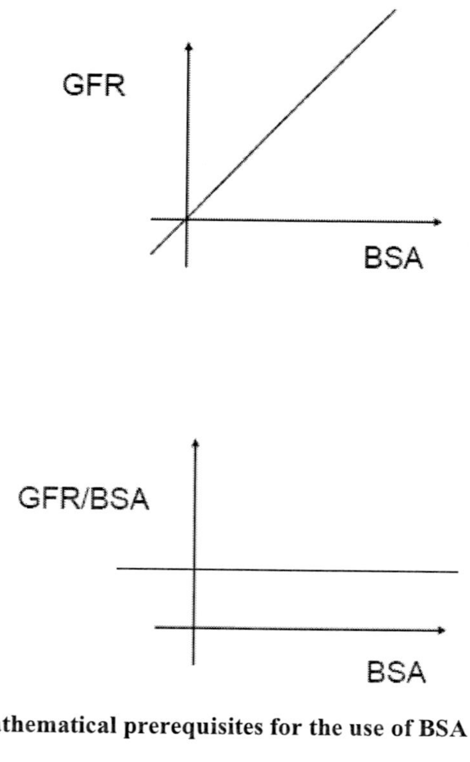

Figure 1. Illustration of mathematical prerequisites for the use of BSA indexing.

Indexing GFR and using ratio as size adjustment is largely debated in the mathematical and statistical literature. As mathematical demonstrations are often complicated for medical doctors (including us!), this type of articles is largely ignored by clinical physicians. However, their conclusions are concordant and all authors publishing on ratio as size adjustment talk of "spurious correlation"[5,6,9,20]. In 1949, Tanner already explained these theoretical arguments against the use of BSA indexing [5]. Tanner's article was cited by H.W. Smith in his famous physiological book published in 1951 (The kidney: structure and function in health and disease). In his reference book, Smith accepted the BSA indexation. Nevertheless, the author himself did not seem very convinced by the existing arguments that he described in only two pages. He wrote: "...the writer believes that the surface area basis comparison *cannot be improved* upon at the present time. This decision is affirmed despite the Tanner's criticism"[25].

Why such success? Or the consequences of indexing for BSA

The success of the BSA indexation and the absence of calling into question of such a use are linked to the simplicity (simpleness?) of its use on the one hand and the absence of consequences of this indexation on GFR results in global populations on the other hand [1]. Indeed, as we have illustrated it in Table 1, indexing GFR for BSA has very limited consequences in "normal" body size patients [1,3,26]. If indexing GFR for BSA is negligible in normal body size people, consequences on GFR results will be important and clinically significant in obese or anorectic patients [1,3]. Once again, this fact is illustrated in Table 1.

Table 1. Mean differences between absolute (ml/min) and indexed (ml/min/1,73m^2) GFR (* = $p<0.0001$). BMI in kg/m^2. "Reproduced with the permission of Oxford University Press"[1]

	N	Mean absolute GFR	Mean indexed GFR (Du Bois)	Mean difference between indexed GFR (Du Bois) and absolute GFR
BMI 18,5 – 25	40	44.47	43.38	-1.09
BMI over 30	81	98.55	81.73	-18.2 *
BMI over 40	33	110.17	87.76	-24.85 *

When McIntosh or Smith was writing, obesity was rare (at least compared to now) and obese patients were relatively rarely studied. One can understand the relatively poor attention H.W. Smith had accorded to BSA indexation as this indexation permitted comparison between populations without clinically significant modification of a specific patient's result [25]. Today, obesity is epidemic in Western countries [27]. In such obese patients, indexing absolute GFR for BSA strongly modifies the final results and this can have huge consequences for example in the dosage adaptation of nephrotoxic drugs [3,28-30]. For some therapy (notably in oncology), the treatment dosage is also determined from the BSA patient (but this is very questionable regarding pharmacokinetic studies, see [30-32]).

This, once again, will have implications especially in obese or anorectic patients [3,22,29-31,33,34], as this has been especially well illustrated by Felici and Verbraecken [29,31]. The question of the validity of BSA indexation is thus topical (not only in Nephrology) and insisting on the weakness of this indexation still makes sense at the beginning of the 21st century.

The "1.73m²" Value: The Other Icon

As we have already mentioned, the choice of the number 1.73 m² was proposed by McIntosh in 1928 [10]. It was based on population data published by Fisk in 1923 [35]. At this time, the mean BSA of the population studied was 1.72 m² (which became 1.73 m² by error (*sic*) as recently suggested by Heaf [36]). This population was not really representative of the American population as these data were obtained in young citizens 25 years old applying for life insurance [35]. Height and weight measurements were not free from criticisms because subjects were clothed and authors subtracted 1 inch from height for shoes and 5 pounds from weight for clothes for women (1.5 inches and 4 pounds for men)[36]. As Smith *et al* already underlined in 1951, the choice of 1.73 m² is totally arbitrary. This author compiled weight and height of patients included in 11 study teams involved in GFR measurement. From these 263 men and 164 women, the calculated BSA was 1.83 and 1.81 m², respectively. As 1.73 m² was already used in innumerable data and because it was thought important that each author used the same number, Smith *et al* accepted 1.73 m² [25]. In 2007, Heaf [36] elegantly illustrated that the choice of 1.73 m² was, retrospectively, probably not the best using anthropometrical data published in vast American and European recent statistical reports [37,38]. It is well known that the mean weight in the global population has increased in the last decades, especially in the USA [27]. Compared to the 1.73m², the numbers proposed by Heaf are not surprisingly higher, i.e. 1.92 m² in USA and 1.86 m² in Europe [36]. However, we agree with Smith's argument. The choice of 1.73 as the reference is arbitrary and thus not the most important. The most important is that everybody uses the same reference. Even so, choosing such a so low value (in the light of the current "heavy" population) will have the strongest consequences in the indexation results of obese patients and we have already illustrated that BSA indexation has the more important consequences in this kind of patients [1,3].

How to Estimate BSA: The "Mythic" Du Bois' Equation and Other "Magic" Equations

BSA is the classical anthropometric data which is the most difficult (for the subject and the researcher) to measure directly [4,28,39-41]. Very few authors have in fact directly measured BSA in the last decades (the most recent technique consists of covering body with alginate, a fine powder that hardens with water but remains soft, like rubber gloves (it is used in artificial teeth))[28,42]. Some authors have even suggested that such a measure is impossible because related to the “ruler” used for its measurement. For example, the measurement of the Britain coast will vary with the size of the “ruler” used: the smaller the ruler, the longer the length (if an infinitesimally small ruler is used, the length of the Britain coast may be infinite!). *Sensu strico,* the same reasoning can be made for BSA measurement regarding the microscopic features of the skin [36,43,44]. Whatever, we may ask why such a difficult measurable data seemed so important for scientists at the end of the 19th and at the beginning of the 20th century. In fact, BSA was thought to be the best predictor (but we know now it is not true [4,6]) of BMR which was also difficult to measure directly. As BSA has been early thought to be estimated from height and weight (or from any other easy measurable data), several authors had studied different ways to estimate BSA [44-46]. One major work on this topic already published in 1879 by Meeh, proposed an estimating equation based only on weight [47]. However, in this field, the most famous BSA equation based on weight and height was published in 1916 by Du Bois and Du Bois (spelt DuBois in [45] and Du Bois in [48]) [48]. Because this equation is still largely used nowadays, it seems to us interesting to focus on this publication. The reference method to measure BSA (in most but not all patients) was ingenious and merits recall. Clothed patients’ bodies were covered with moulds of gummed manila paper (a kind of tailor’s paper). The moulds were cut open, placed flat on photographic paper which was then exposed to sunlight. The unexposed paper was cut and weighed. Knowing the density area of the photographic area, BSA was deduced. The authors did the following precisions in their article: the head was covered and the nose was covered the last and two holes were left to breath through; hands are difficult to cover with such paper and hard paraffin was used over thin cotton gloves; areas back of the ears, skin between the toes, penis and scrotum (*sic*) were geometrically determined; lastly, only very small portions of the face and ears (eye-sockets and concavities of the ear) were not measured!! [45,48,49]. The Du Bois brothers first studied five patients and derived a geometrical formula estimating BSA with measurements of 7 parts of the body (19 measurements in all)(Table 2)[45]. Correlation with direct measurement was excellent and this geometrical formula is still now considered as a reference method by most authors but is nearly never used because it is cumbersome [44,45,50,51]. One year later, the same brothers published, in the same journal, a formula to estimate BSA only based on weight and height, which can be seen as easier to apply [48]. To their five initial patients, they added four others. Among this population of 9 patients, there was a 2-year-old child suffering from rickets weighting 6.27 kg, one obese female (100 kg for 1.50 m), one 36-year-old subject with mental and physical development of a boy of 8 (24.2 kg for 1.1 m), and an 18-year-old subject with type 1 diabetes (treated with whisky to block gluconeogenesis!) and low weight (45.25 kg)[48,49]. Two legless cripples were also included at the origin but were excluded from the final analysis (*sic*) [49]. Du Bois and Du Bois then developed a formula based on weight and height for BSA estimation with this very limited and very heterogeneous sample (Table 2). The mean error with their formula was 1.5% (maximum 5%) in their subjects [48]. Numerous criticisms were expressed notably concerning mathematical and statistical methods used, but one must keep in mind that, at that time, all calculations were made “by hand” [1,8,51,52]. Regarding statistical and methodological limitations (limited number of patients, extraordinary heterogeneous population), the most astonishing fact is that this estimation equation does not work so bad [29,33,39-41,44,51-54]!!

Table 2. Geometrical (or "linear") formula for calculating BSA. BSA is generated by the addition of the seven values obtained (taken with subject lying on a flat surface) [45]

Head	AB X 0.308	A = around vertex and point of chin B = coronal circumference around occiput and forehead, just above eyebrows
Arms	F(G+H+I) X 0.611	F = tip of acromial process to lower border of radius, measured with extended G = circumference at level of upper border of axilla H = largest circumference of forearm (just below elbow) I = smallest circumference of forearm (just above head of ulna)
Hands	JK X 2.22	J = lower posterior border of radius to tip of second finger K = circumference of open hand at the meta-carpo-phalangeal joints
Trunk	L(M+N) X 0.703	L = suprasternal notch to upper border of pubes M = circumference of abdomen at level of umbilicus N = circumference of thorax at level of nipples in the male and just above breasts in the female
Thighs	O(P+Q) X 0.508	O = superior border of great trochanter to the lower border of the patella P = circumference of thigh just below the level of perineum Q = circumference of hips and buttocks at the level of the great trochanters
Legs	RS X 1.4	R = from sole of foot to lower border of patella S = circumference at level of lower border of patella
Feet	T(U+V) X 1.04	T = length of foot including great toe U = circumference of foot at base of little toe V = smallest circumference of hankle (just above malleoli)

Table 3. Most used formulas based on weight and height to estimate BSA (weight in kg, height in cm and BSA in m^2)

Authors	Formula	Number of patients studied	Ref
Du Bois and Du Bois	0.007184 X weight$^{0.425}$ X height$^{0.725}$	9	[48]
Boyd	0.01788 X weight$^{0.484}$ X height$^{0.5}$	197	[57]
Gehan and George	0.0235 X weight$^{0.51456}$ X height$^{0.42246}$	401	[40]
Haycock *et al*	0.024265 X weight$^{0.5378}$ X height$^{0.3964}$	81	[55]
Mosteller	(weight$^{0.5}$ X height$^{0.5}$)/60	non determined	[56]
Livingston *et al*	0.1173 X weight$^{0.6466}$	45	[50]

Indeed, several authors have proposed other formulas studying larger populations with best statistical methods (Table 3) but with no clear practical advantage over the Du Bois' formula (except for subjects with weight under 10 kg where Haycock [55] or Mosteller [56] formulas are preferred). In fact, all the formulas give more or less the same results even if they seem very different [29,33,40-42,53,54].

This is not a new miracle. Indeed, Bailey has elegantly demonstrated that in all equations weight and height are strongly correlated [41]. Populations studied by different authors having built these equations are in fact comparable in term of body size. For example in the 401 subjects studied by Gehan and Georges (probably the best equation from a statistical and methodological points of view with data from the largest historical cohort published by Boyd in 1935 [57]), only two subjects had BMI over 30 kg/m² (and Gehan's equation strongly misestimates BSA at least in one of these patients)[40]. In the non-obese population, it is clear that height and weight are strictly linked (the taller the patient is, the heavier he is)[39,41,54]. On this way, it seems logical that all the BSA estimating equations are comparable in the normal body size population (and all these equations could be replaced by equations with only one variable, height or weight! [41,42,44,50]). For the obese patients, such reasoning is not applicable because in these subjects, gain of weight is not linked to gain of height (but especially linked to gain of abdominal circumference). In mathematical terms, obese patients can be seen as "spherical" although normal body size patients are "cylindric"[41,52]. As sphere is the volume with the lowest surface, one can presume that BSA estimation in obese calculated from an equation built from a "cylindric" non obese population will overestimate true BSA [40,41]. As we have already said, measuring BSA is not easy and this is even more problematic in obese subject [50]. For this reason, very few studies have directly measured BSA in obese patients. To the best of our knowledge, only Tucker and Alexander measured BSA in obese patients but this population included only 4 subjects. These authors showed that the Du Bois equation was not accurate in these patients. Moreover, they also underlined that the first linear formula from Du Bois also overestimates measured BSA and it was logically explained by the error induced by the measurement of the trunk and thighs in these patients (now these two area are 50 to 65% of the total BSA)[58]. Du Bois and Gehan had themselves underlined the probable inaccuracy of their linear formula for obese patients [40,48]. In 2001, Livingston proposed a new equation specifically for obese patients (logically built only from weight) but unfortunately, BSA was not directly measured and the Du Bois linear equation remained considered as the reference, which is a non sense [1,50]. In 2006, Verbraecken compared BSA results from 7 different equations in 1868 patients [29]. Among these, there were 757 obese subjects included. Unfortunately, the interest of this study is limited because BSA was not directly measured. The mean BSA result from the seven equations was however considered as the reference. The authors have chosen the mean "because the 7 formulas have all been derived in independent studies and the mean of any available independent estimates is the best measure". However, this last assertion is not correct as the Mosteller's, the Boyd's and the Gehan-Georges's equations have been derived from the same cohort. Whatever, in the non obese population, the authors confirmed that all formulas give more or less the same results. In obese patients, strong conclusions are impossible in the absence of true BSA measurement. The authors can only conclude that mean BSA is higher in obese population versus non obese population (not a revolutionary finding indeed!) and that the results from the Mosteller's equations are higher than from the Du Bois's and lower than the Gehan's formula in obese patients. The authors finally wrote: "Moreover, we do not really know which is the exact BSA…With obesity, weight increases without a proportional increase in height. Consequently, it is possible that the Du Bois-type predicting formulas…could systematically miscalculate BSA for obese patients" [29]. This was already the theory advanced by Bailey [41], so Verbraecken's study does not add any new information.

To close this chapter on BSA equations, it is interesting to note that some authors have recently described new methods for BSA measuring with body three dimensions scans. However, these methods are not perfect (notably for the obese because of the skin folds), costly and source of irradiation [28,59].

Indexing GFR for BSA in Abnormal Body Size Subjects: Reductio Ad Absurdum

Several theoretical arguments do exist against the use of BSA indexing [1]. The inadequacy of such use is however difficult to describe in normal body size population because, once again, indexation has nearly no consequences on GFR results. We have thus studied two different abnormal body size populations i.e. obese and anorectic (anorexia nervosa) patients. We will use the topic of estimating GFR by creatinine based equations (and specially the MDRD study equation) (Table 4) to illustrate, *reductio ad absurdum,* our hypothesis [60,61].

Table 4. The MDRD study equation

4-variable MDRD Study equation

GFR (mL/min/1.73m^2) = 175 x SCr (mg/dL) $^{-1.154}$ x Age $^{-0.203}$ x 0.742 (if woman)

X 1.21 for Black-American
X 0.763 for Japanese
X 1,233 for Chinese

Firstly, GFR and creatinine have been measured in 100 obese patients. Of these 100 patients, only patients with measured GFR over 60 mL/min/1.73m^2 were considered for our purpose (n=81). Most of these patients were hospitalized for slimming courses. They were frankly obese as their mean weight and BMI were 113±28 kg (range: 76 to 258 kg) and 41±9 kg/m^2, respectively. Mean absolute GFR was 101±24 mL/min (measured with the plasma clearance of Cr-EDTA [62]) although mean indexed GFR was 76±16 mL/min/1.73m^2 (mean difference between absolute and indexed: 25±14 mL/min). Mean serum creatinine (measured with an IDMS traceable method) was 0.80±0.23 mg/dL. Estimated GFR with the MDRD study equation in this population was 90±22 mL/min/1.73m². If absolute GFR is used as the reference, MDRD study equation underestimates measured GFR (mean difference: -11±20 mL/min). If the indexed GFR is used as the reference, the MDRD equation overestimates measured GFR (mean difference: +14±18 mL/min/1.73m²)(Table 5).

Table 5. Bias induced by the MDRD study equation in an obese population with GFR indexed by BSA or not

	Mean difference between MDRD and indexed GFR	Mean difference between MDRD and absolute GFR
Obesity (n=81, GFR over 60 ml/min)	+14 ± 18 mL/min/1.73m²	-11 ± 20 mL/min

Using indexed GFR as reference, the MDRD study equation will overestimate GFR results in our obese population. Although obese, all the patients included have a measured GFR above 60 mL/min. From several studies, it can be concluded that the MDRD study equation systematically underestimates GFR in healthy subjects (and in subjects with "normal" or "near normal" creatinine levels). This GFR underestimation by the MDRD study equation is explained by several factors (notably the fact that this equation has been built from a chronic kidney disease population)[60,63,64]. There are absolutely no good reasons to believe that this well-established underestimation in low creatinine values does not occur in the obese population. In the same way, there is no reason to believe that the creatinine-based MDRD equation overestimates measured GFR in this population, as it is the case when indexed GFR is considered. GFR underestimation by the MDRD equation is only found in our obese patients when absolute GFR measurements are used.

Another example can be done with the other "extreme population", i.e. anorectic patients [65]. GFR was systematically measured in twenty seven patients. As expected, the population was young (30 ± 13 years old) and very thin (mean weight: 42 ± 7 kg, mean BMI: 15 ± 2 kg/m²). Mean measured GFR was 68 ± 23 mL/min and the GFR range was large (13 to 134 ml/min) if absolute GFR was used. In this very specific population, serum creatinine has a very poor sensitivity to detect GFR under 60 ml/min/1.73 m² (56% of sensibility which means that one anorectic patient over two will have kidney disease with serum creatinine in the normal range). In the same way, the MDRD study equation will strongly overestimate measured GFR in this population (+39 ± 39 mL/min). These two results are not surprising because serum creatinine concentration is largely dependent on muscular mass, as creatinine is the catabolite of the muscular protein creatine. Because anorectic patients have, of course, a decreased muscular mass, their serum creatinine will not rise as expected in renal failure. We are showing now our results when indexed GFR for BSA is used in place of absolute GFR. In this condition, mean indexed GFR is logically higher (80 mL/min/1.73 m²). The creatinine sensitivity (determined by ROC curves) to detect GFR under 60 mL/min/1.73m² is striking. Indeed, sensitivity of serum creatinine would be of 75%. Based on the well known creatinine sensitivity in the global population, sensitivity of creatinine in this very low muscular mass population could be seen as good (or even better) than in the "normal" body size population [65,66]. This is of course a non-sense, once again induced by the use of the BSA indexation.

Indexing GFR for BSA: Data from Comparative Physiology: The Mouse and the Elephant

We have thus exposed all the limitations of BSA indexing. However, it also seems logical that mice GFR can't be directly compared with elephants GFR. We can take this last affirmation at its word and take arguments from comparative physiology. Singer has recently compiled and compared data from veterinary literature [67,68]. Of course, measuring BSA in elephants or pigs is not easy and most studies have measured GFR and weight. As it is shown in Singer's review article, relationship does exist between GFR and weight when different animals are compared (Figure 2). However, this relationship is not linear but well exponential. In other words, if the horse weight is 16000 times higher than the mouse weight (30 g versus 500 kg), the horse GFR is only 4000 times higher than the mouse GFR [67]. Once again, if we restrict the analysis in the limits of the human race, relation between GFR and weight (or BSA) would appear non-linear and indexing GFR by BSA will be thus misleading.

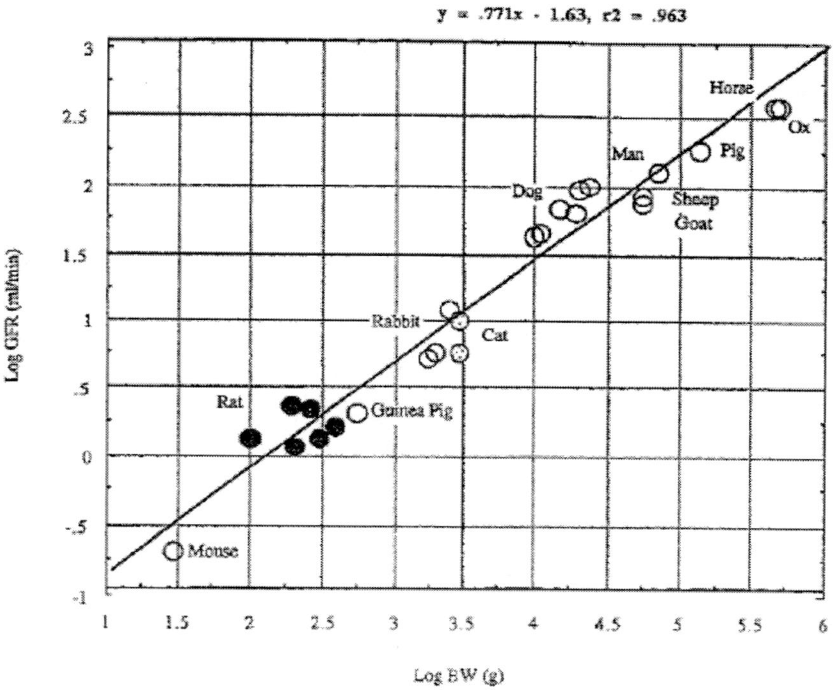

Figure 2. Logarithmic relationship between GFR and weight in 12 species of mammals. "Reprinted from Am J Kidney Dis , 35, Singer MA, Morton AR, Mouse to elephant: biological scaling and Kt/V , 306-309, 2000, with permission from Elsevier" [67].

Comparing absolute and indexed GFR in obese and non obese subjects will have relatively low impact on the results, compared to the impact of the indexation for mice and elephants' GFR values [67,68]. If weight is not the best way, another indexation must be found [67]. Once again based on the Singer's review work, the true physiological indexation could be BMR. Indeed, BMR and GFR have the same relationship to weight (exponent 0.75)[67,68]. Moreover, from animal studies regarding the effect of changing BMR (for example inducing hypothyroidism or studying hibernating animals), it could be stated that BMR is the primary process that sets GFR (as other physiological functions as cardiac output and pulmonary functions)[68]. In the Singer's hypothesis, ammonia could be the link, the messenger and the regulator between BMR and GFR (see [69] for more details). One major proof of the central role of BMR is the ratio of GFR to BMR which is fully independent of size and is constant in all animals (from reptiles to mammals reflecting its importance of this design rule since it has been well conserved from an evolutionary perspective)[67-69]. The optimal GFR can be defined by this ratio by each unit of metabolic rate. As BMR also influences body size, GFR and body size are interdependent but body size does not set GFR [67,68]. The pivotal role of BMR had already been suggested by Holten in 1931 and some other authors (see below)[11,70,71]. Of course, this theory, even if very interesting from an intellectual point of view, is of relatively poor interest in humans because BMR is very difficult to measure with precision and indexing GFR for BMR will probably have no success in practice.

Other Ways to Index GFR: Some Perspectives

Several authors are convinced of limitations linked to BSA indexation and have thus proposed other ways to index GFR. One of the most evoked factors to index GFR in obese patients is height, a very easy measurable variable. Two studies have shown that corrected GFR (or renal plasma flow) for height is identical in obese and non obese ("nephrologically" normal) populations whereas corrected GFR for BSA is inadequately lower in obese population [72,73]. However, we have already criticized this kind of argument (i.e. lowering dispersion of data). As the range of height in the population is narrower than the range of weight (giants and dwarves are less numerous than obese or anorectic), it is logical that indexing for height will decreases dispersion of data in adult population. But it is not sufficient. Indeed, the fundamental prerequisite relation between GFR and height (and the lack of relation between GFR indexed for height and height) has not been studied. Moreover, normal values for GFR indexed for height remain to be determined and could be artificially different in men and women (because men are taller). The same limitations can be advanced for the use of lean body mass [70,72,74] or ideal body weight [75], which both are strongly (and only) dependent of height (and it is now important to recall that McIntosh in the *princeps* article on this topic used ideal weight and not current "true" weight [10]). Moreover ideal and lean body mass are calculated from weight which will appears two times in the same formula. For all these reasons, we think that correcting GFR for height or "weight shunt from height" [75] is not indicated.

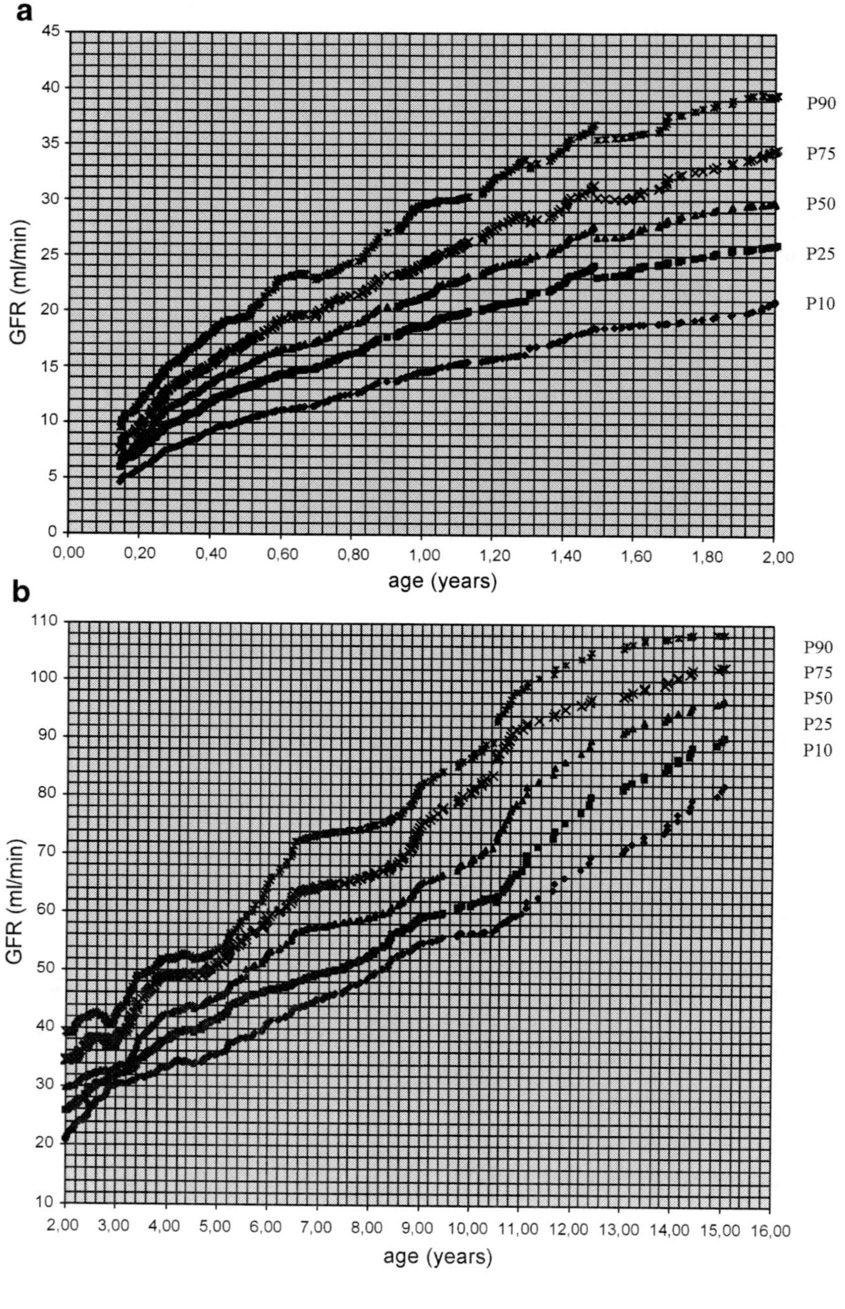

Figure 3. The 10th, 25th, 50th, 75th and 90th percentile curves of normal Cr-EDTA clearance values, not corrected for body surface area, in function of age from 623 children. a: 0.1 to 2 years, b: 2 to 15 years "With kind permission from Springer Science+Business Media: Eur J Nucl Med Mol Imaging Escaping the correction for body surface area when calculating glomerular filtration rate in children 2008 , Piepsz A, Tondeur M, Ham H, Figure 1,"[92].

Some authors proposed that GFR must be indexed with total body water (TBW) [26,76] or extracellular volume fluid (ECFV)[8,26,77,78]. Indeed, it seems intuitively better to correct GFR for ECFV or TBW because one of the roles of the kidney is to regulate body fluid composition. Nevertheless, ECFV are not so easy to measure (and TBW even more difficult [26]). Indexing GFR for ECFV could only be done when GFR is measured with urinary clearance [79,80] (because measure of ECFV is then considered as equivalent to the volume of distribution of the GFR marker used)[80]. Moreover, mathematical prerequisites have been poorly studied. Peters *et al* argue that using ECFV indexing had excellent reproducibility on GFR measurement [81], and makes GFR "normal" values identical in male and women [77,80] and in young infants and adults (GFR in infancy could even be higher) [26,78]. However, once again, all these "proofs" are indirect [82]. Even with these limitations and even if indexing for ECFV is still using a ratio and is thus "mathematically" questionable [5,9], we agree with these authors: indexing GFR for ECFV is of interest and we need additional researches on this topic [1].

As other authors, we suggest that the only way to harmonise data and determine normal values is to use regression analysis on large population sample with different age, sex and body size [1,5,6,20,21]. This work needs a multicentric study because a large sample is needed but, as Turner *et al* have said "only when this is done will the physician who examines one patient at a time also be able to abandon the practice of indexing"[6]. In cardiology, such a work has been done for cardiac dimensions (of course, much easier to measure than GFR) and had confirmed the lack of interest of simple indexation favouring correction with allometric exponent of weight [83,84]. In Nephrology, the recent study published by Piepsz [79] in paediatric population is of the greatest interest, too. In children, age is clearly the most important variable to establish GFR reference values. These authors have thus elaborated age-related percentiles of absolute GFR in their large population of paediatric healthy subjects using absolute GFR. GFR was measured by a reference method (Cr-EDTA). Such tables are easy to use in daily practice and avoid difficulties linked to BSA indexation (Figure 3)[79].

In absence of definitive arguments in favour of one or another indexation in the adult population, we propose to use non-indexed, absolute GFR [1].

Conclusions

There are several strong limitations to the use of GFR indexation with BSA. This indexation could effectively be seen as a myth. Indeed, it is based on very poor physiological data. Its application is often implicit, blind, and nearly unconscious.

Applying BSA indexation has nearly no effect on GFR results in the normal body size population. So why still to use it?

Applying BSA indexation has more numerical effect in "abnormal" body size population. This effect is probably largely overestimated. Moreover, the estimation of BSA by classical equations is neither precise nor accurate, just in this obese population where indexing for BSA has real impact. So why still to use it?

To end this polemic chapter, we will take words from McCance who criticized BSA indexation (in favour of TBW) in 1952. The sentence may be viewed as pessimist but is (unfortunately from our point of view) realist, retrospectively: "Even in the so-called objective sciences any proposals involving changes in established thought or practice are likely to meet with considerable opposition…It is hoped nevertheless that our suggestions will receive at least some objective consideration"[76]. Indeed, if many physiologists, especially those involved in the renal physiology of obese patients, have well integrated the BSA indexation weakness and notably the impact on the obesity-associated glomerular hyperfiltration [85-91], most of clinical physicians and clinical researchers (even in the obesity field) are still using this misleading indexation.

References

[1] Delanaye P, Radermecker RP, Rorive M, Depas G, Krzesinski JM (2005) Indexing glomerular filtration rate for body surface area in obese patients is misleading: concept and example. *Nephrol. Dial. Transplant.* 20:2024-2028.

[2] Mathew TH (2005) Chronic kidney disease and automatic reporting of estimated glomerular filtration rate: a position statement. *Med. J. Aust.* 183:138-141.

[3] Lamb EJ, Tomson CR, Roderick PJ (2005) Estimating kidney function in adults using formulae. *Ann. Clin. Biochem*. 42:321-345.

[4] Krovetz LJ (1965). The physiologic significance of body surface area. *J. Pediatr.* 67:841-862.

[5] Tanner JM (1949) Fallacy of per-weight and per-surface area standards, and their relation to spurious correlation. *J. Appl. Physiol.* 2:1-15.

[6] Turner ST, Reilly SL (1995) Fallacy of indexing renal and systemic hemodynamic measurements for body surface area. *Am. J. Physiol.* 268:R978-R988.

[7] Rubin MI, Bruck E, Rapoport (1949) Maturation of renal function in childhood; clearance studies. *J. Clin. Invest* 28:1144-1162.

[8] White AJ, Strydom WJ (1991) Normalisation of glomerular filtration rate measurements. *Eur. J. Nucl. Med.* 18:385-390.

[9] Kronmal RA (1993) Spurious correlation and the fallacy of the ratio standard revisited. *J. R. Statist. Soc. A.* 156:379-392.

[10] McIntosh JF, Möller R, Van Slycke DD (1928) Studies on urea excretions. III. The influence of body size on urea outpout. *J. Clin. Invest* 6:467-483.

[11] Holten C (1931) The dependence of the normal kidney function on the size of the body. *Acta Paediatr. Stock.* 12:251-267.

[12] Taylor FB, Drury DR, Addis T (1923) The regulation of renal activity. The relation between the rate of urea excretion and the size of the kidneys. *Am. J. Physiol.* 65:55-61.

[13] Stewart GN (1921) Possible relations of the weight of the lungs and other organs to body-weight and surface area (in dogs). *Am. J. Physiol.* 58:45-52.

[14] MacKay EM (1932) Kidney weight, body size and renal function. *Arch. Intern. Med.* 50:590-594.

[15] McCance RA, Young WF (1941) The secretion of urine by newborn infants. *J. Physiol.* 99:265-282.

[16] Barnett HL, Hare K, (1948) Measurement of glomerular filtration rate in premature infants. *J. Clin. Invest* 27:691-699.

[17] Dean RF, McCance RA (1947) Inulin, diodone, creatinine and urea clearances in newborn infants. *J. Physiol.* 106:431-439.

[18] Gordon HH, Harrison HE, McNamara H (1942) The urea clearance of young premature and full term infants. *J. Clin. Invest* 21:499-504.

[19] Schoenthal L, Lurie D, Kelly M (1933) Urea clearance in normal and in dehydrated infants. Renal function in intestinal intoxication. *Am. J. Dis. Child* 45:41-53.

[20] Albrecht GH, Gelvin BR, Hartman SE (1993) Ratios as a size adjustment in morphometrics. *Am. J. Phys. Anthropol.* 91:441-468.

[21] Watson WS (2000) Body surface area correction in single-sample methods of glomerular filtration rate estimation. *Nucl. Med. Commun.* 21:121-122.

[22] Dooley MJ, Poole SG (2000) Poor correlation between body surface area and glomerular filtration rate. *Cancer Chemother. Pharmacol.* 46:523-526.

[23] Morgan DB, Dillon S, Payne RB (1978) The assessment of glomerular function: creatinine clearance or plasma creatinine? *Postgrad. Med. J.* 54:302-310.

[24] Nyengaard JR, Bendtsen TF (1992) Glomerular number and size in relation to age, kidney weight, and body surface in normal man. *Anat. Rec.* 232:194-201.

[25] Smith H. *The kidney: Structure and function in health and disease*. New York, 1951.

[26] Bird NJ, Henderson BL, Lui D, Ballinger JR, Peters AM (2003) Indexing glomerular filtration rate to suit children. *J. Nucl. Med.* 44:1037-1043.

[27] Flegal KM (2005) Epidemiologic aspects of overweight and obesity in the United States. *Physiol. Behav.* 86:599-602.

[28] Lee JY, Choi JW (2006) Validity and reliability of an alginate method to measure body surface area. *J. Physiol. Anthropol.* 25:247-255.

[29] Verbraecken J, Van de HP, De Backer W, Van Gaal L (2006) Body surface area in normal-weight, overweight, and obese adults. A comparison study. *Metabolism* 55:515-524.

[30] Kaestner SA, Sewell GJ (2007) Chemotherapy dosing part I: scientific basis for current practice and use of body surface area. *Clin. Oncol.* 19:23-37.

[31] Felici A, Verweij J, Sparreboom A (2002) Dosing strategies for anticancer drugs: the good, the bad and body-surface area. *Eur. J. Cancer* 38:1677-1684.

[32] Grochow LB, Baraldi C, Noe D (1990) Is dose normalization to weight or body surface area useful in adults? *J. Natl. Cancer Inst.* 82:323-325.

[33] van der Sijs H., Guchelaar HJ (2002) Formulas for calculating body surface area. *Ann. Pharmacother.* 36:345-346.

[34] Hunter RJ, Navo MA, Thaker PH, Bodurka DC, Wolf JK, Smith JA (2009) Dosing chemotherapy in obese patients: Actual versus assigned body surface area (BSA). *Cancer Treat. Rev.* 35:69-78.

[35] Fisk EL, Crawford JR. *How to make the periodic health examination*. New York, 1927; 345.

[36] Heaf JG (2007). The origin of the 1 x 73-m2 body surface area normalization: problems and implications. *Clin. Physiol. Funct. Imaging* 27:135-137.
[37] Health Satistics. Key data on health. Office for official publications of the european community, Luxembourg, 2002; 146.
[38] Ogden CL, Fryar CD, Carroll MD, Flegal KM (2004) *Mean body weight, height, and body mass index*, United States 1960-2002. Adv Data1-17.
[39] Sendroy J, Jr., Cecchini LP (1954) Determination of human body surface area from height and weight. *J. Appl. Physiol.* 7:1-12.
[40] Gehan EA, George SL (1970) Estimation of human body surface area from height and weight. *Cancer Chemother. Rep.* 54:225-235.
[41] Bailey BJ, Briars GL (1996) Estimating the surface area of the human body. *Stat. Med.* 15:1325-1332.
[42] Lee JY, Choi JW, Kim H (2008) Determination of body surface area and formulas to estimate body surface area using the alginate method. *J. Physiol. Anthropol.* 27:71-82.
[43] Slone TH (1993) Body surface area misconceptions. *Risk Anal.* 13:375-377.
[44] Gibson S, Numa A (2003) The importance of metabolic rate and the folly of body surface area calculations. *Anaesthesia* 58:50-55.
[45] Dubois D, DuBois EF (1915) The measurement of the surface area of man. *Arch. Intern. Med.* 16:868-881.
[46] Rubner M (1883) Ueber den einfluss der körpergrösse auf stoff- und draftwechsel. Z. *Biol.* 19:535-562.
[47] Meeh K (1879) Oberflächenmessungen des menschlichen Körpers. *Z. Biol.* 15:425-458.
[48] Dubois D, Dubois E (1916) A formula to estimate the approximative surface area if height and weight be known. *Arch. Intern. Med.* 17:863-871.
[49] Sawyer M, Stone RH, Du Bois EF (1916) Further measurements of the surface area of adults and children. *Arch. Intern. Med.* 17:855-862.
[50] Livingston EH, Lee S (2001) Body surface area prediction in normal-weight and obese patients. *Am. J. Physiol. Endocrinol. Metab.* 281:E586-E591.
[51] Shuter B, Aslani A (2000) Body surface area: Du Bois and Du Bois revisited. *Eur. J. Appl. Physiol.* 82:250-254.
[52] Burton RF (2008) Estimating body surface area from mass and height: theory and the formula of Du Bois and Du Bois. *Ann. Hum. Biol.* 35:170-184.
[53] Reading BD, Freeman B (2005) Simple formula for the surface area of the body and a simple model for anthropometry. *Clin. Anat.* 18:126-130.
[54] Blake GM, Grewal GS (2005) An evaluation of the body surface area correction for 51Cr-EDTA measurements of glomerular filtration rate. *Nucl. Med. Commun.* 26:447-451.
[55] Haycock GB, Schwartz GJ, Wisotsky DH (1978) Geometric method for measuring body surface area: a height-weight formula validated in infants, children, and adults. *J. Pediatr.* 93:62-66.
[56] Mosteller RD (1987) Simplified calculation of body-surface area. *N. Engl. J. Med.* 317:1098.
[57] Boyd E. The growth of the Surface of the Human Body. Minneapolis, 1935.

[58] Tucker GR, Alexander JK (1960) Estimation of body surface area of extremely obese human subjects. *J. Appl. Physiol.* 15:781-784.

[59] Tikuisis P, Meunier P, Jubenville CE (2001) Human body surface area: measurement and prediction using three dimensional body scans. *Eur. J. Appl. Physiol.* 85:264-271.

[60] Delanaye P, Cohen EP (2008) Formula-based estimates of the GFR: equations variable and uncertain. *Nephron Clin. Pract.* 110:c48-c53.

[61] Levey AS, Bosch JP, Lewis JB, Greene T, Rogers N, Roth D (1999) A more accurate method to estimate glomerular filtration rate from serum creatinine: a new prediction equation. Modification of Diet in Renal Disease Study Group. *Ann. Intern. Med.* 130:461-470.

[62] Brandstrom E, Grzegorczyk A, Jacobsson L, Friberg P, Lindahl A, Aurell M (1998) GFR measurement with iohexol and 51Cr-EDTA. A comparison of the two favoured GFR markers in Europe. *Nephrol. Dial. Transplant.* 13:1176-1182.

[63] Froissart M, Rossert J, Jacquot C, Paillard M, Houillier P (2005) Predictive performance of the modification of diet in renal disease and Cockcroft-Gault equations for estimating renal function. *J. Am. Soc. Nephrol.* 16:763-773.

[64] Delanaye P, Cavalier E, Krzesinski JM, Chapelle JP (2006) Why the MDRD equation should not be used in patients with normal renal function (and normal creatinine values)? *Clin. Nephrol.* 66:147-148.

[65] Delanaye P, Cavalier E, Radermecker RP, Paquot N, Depas G, Chapelle JP, Scheen AJ, Krzesinski JM (2008) Cystatin C or Creatinine for Detection of Stage 3 Chronic Kidney Disease in Anorexia Nervosa. *Nephron Clin. Pract.* 110:c158-c163.

[66] Couchoud C, Pozet N, Labeeuw M, Pouteil-Noble C (1999) Screening early renal failure: cut-off values for serum creatinine as an indicator of renal impairment. *Kidney Int.* 55:1878-1884.

[67] Singer MA, Morton AR (2000) Mouse to elephant: biological scaling and Kt/V. Am. J. *Kidney Dis.* 35:306-309.

[68] Singer MA (2001) Of mice and men and elephants: metabolic rate sets glomerular filtration rate. *Am. J. Kidney Dis.* 37:164-178.

[69] Singer MA (2001) Ammonia functions as a regulatory molecule to mediate adjustments in glomerular filtration rate in response to changes in metabolic rate. *Med. Hypotheses* 57:740-744.

[70] Kurtin PS (1988) Standardization of renal function measurements in children: kidney size versus metabolic rate. *Child Nephrol. Urol.* 9:337-339.

[71] Holliday MA. Body composition, metabolism and growth. In: Vernier RL, ed. *Pediatric Nephrology*. WilliamsandWilkins, Baltimore: 1987.

[72] Schmieder RE, Beil AH, Weihprecht H, Messerli FH (1995) How should renal hemodynamic data be indexed in obesity? *J. Am. Soc. Nephrol.* 5:1709-1713.

[73] Anastasio P, Spitali L, Frangiosa A, Molino D, Stellato D, Cirillo E, Pollastro RM, Capodicasa L, Sepe J, Federico P, Gaspare DS (2000) Glomerular filtration rate in severely overweight normotensive humans. *Am. J. Kidney Dis.* 35:1144-1148.

[74] Hallynck TH, Soep HH, Thomis JA, Boelaert J, Daneels R, Dettli L (1981) Should clearance be normalised to body surface or to lean body mass? *Br. J. Clin. Pharmacol.* 11:523-526.

[75] Walser M (1990) Progression of chronic renal failure in man. *Kidney Int.* 37:1195-1210.

[76] McCance RA, Widdowson EM (1952) The correct physiological basis on which to compare infant and adult renal function. *Lancet* 2:860-862.

[77] Peters AM (1992) Expressing glomerular filtration rate in terms of extracellular fluid volume. *Nephrol. Dial. Transplant.* 7:205-210.

[78] Peters AM, Gordon I, Sixt R (1994) Normalization of glomerular filtration rate in children: body surface area, body weight or extracellular fluid volume? *J. Nucl. Med.* 35:438-444.

[79] Piepsz A, Tondeur M, Ham H (2008) Escaping the correction for body surface area when calculating glomerular filtration rate in children. *Eur. J. Nucl. Med. Mol. Imaging* 35:1669-1672.

[80] Visser FW, Muntinga JH, Dierckx RA, Navis G (2008) Feasibility and impact of the measurement of extracellular fluid volume simultaneous with GFR by 125I-iothalamate. *Clin. J. Am. Soc. Nephrol.* 3:1308-1315.

[81] Bird NJ, Peters C, Michell AR, Peters AM (2008) Reproducibilities and responses to food intake of GFR measured with chromium-51-EDTA and iohexol simultaneously and independently in normal subjects. *Nephrol. Dial. Transplant.* 23:1902-1909.

[82] Delanaye P, Cavalier E, Froissart M, Krzesinski JM (2008) Reproducibility of GFR measured by chromium-51-EDTA and iohexol. *Nephrol. Dial. Transplant.* 23:4077-4078.

[83] Neilan TG, Pradhan AD, Weyman AE (2008) Derivation of a size-independent variable for scaling of cardiac dimensions in a normal adult population. *J. Am. Soc. Echocardiogr.* 21:779-785.

[84] Neilan TG, Pradhan AD, King ME, Weyman AE (2009) Derivation of a size-independent variable for scaling of cardiac dimensions in a normal paediatric population. *Eur. J. Echocardiogr.* 10:50-55.

[85] Ribstein J, du CG, Mimran A (1995) Combined renal effects of overweight and hypertension. *Hypertension* 26:610-615.

[86] Macdonald J, Marcora S, Jibani M, Roberts G, Kumwenda M, Glover R, Barron J, Lemmey A (2006) GFR estimation using cystatin C is not independent of body composition. *Am. J. Kidney Dis.* 48:712-719.

[87] Chagnac A, Weinstein T, Korzets A, Ramadan E, Hirsch J, Gafter U (2000) Glomerular hemodynamics in severe obesity. *Am. J. Physiol. Renal. Physiol.* 278:F817-F822.

[88] Chagnac A, Weinstein T, Herman M, Hirsh J, Gafter U, Ori Y (2003) The effects of weight loss on renal function in patients with severe obesity. *J. Am. Soc. Nephrol.* 14:1480-1486.

[89] Henegar JR, Bigler SA, Henegar LK, Tyagi SC, Hall JE (2001) Functional and structural changes in the kidney in the early stages of obesity. *J. Am. Soc. Nephrol.* 12:1211-1217.

[90] Bosma RJ, van der Heide JJ, Oosterop EJ, de Jong PE, Navis G (2004) Body mass index is associated with altered renal hemodynamics in non-obese healthy subjects. *Kidney Int.* 65:259-265.

[91] Navarro-Diaz M, Serra A, Romero R, Bonet J, Bayes B, Homs M, Perez N, Bonal J (2006) Effect of drastic weight loss after bariatric surgery on renal parameters in extremely obese patients: long-term follow-up. *J. Am. Soc. Nephrol.* 17:S213-S217.

[92] Piepsz A, Tondeur M, Ham H (2009) Escaping the correction for body surface area when calculating glomerular filtration rate in children. *Eur. J. Nucl. Med. Mol. Imaging* 36:332-333.

In: Nephrology – Dialysis - Transplantation
Editors: Endre Kruger and Kelemen Hahn

ISBN 978-1-60741-736-1
© 2009 Nova Science Publishers, Inc.

Chapter III

Advances in the Peritoneal Dialysis and Future Prospects

Kook-Hwan Oh* and Curie Ahn
Renal Division, Department of Internal Medicine,
Seoul National University College of Medicine, Seoul, Korea
Transplantation Research Institute, Seoul National University, Seoul, Korea

Abstract

Peritoneal dialysis (PD) has been widely used as one of the major renal replacement therapies for end-stage renal disease (ESRD) patients. A new PD fluid is instilled into the peritoneal cavity via peritoneal catheter after the previously instilled fluid has been drained out. Exchange of solutes and water between the body and the peritoneal fluid occurs during PD. PD system has three major components – 1) peritoneal fluid compartment, 2) peritoneal microcirculation and 3) peritoneal membrane. Basic mechanism employed in PD lies in diffusion and convection for removing uremic toxins, and ultrafiltration (UF) for water removal. PD fluid contains a high concentration of glucose, which generates an osmotic gradient between the peritoneal fluid and peritoneal microcirculation, resulting in water movement into the peritoneal cavity. There is a wide inter-individual variation in the speed of solute and water transport through the peritoneal membrane. Peritoneal equilibration test (PET) and other tests for the assessment of the peritoneal solute and water transport have been developed. Fast transporters are likely to dissipate osmotic gradient earlier than slow transporters because they absorb glucose more rapidly through the peritoneal membrane. Suspected factors determining the peritoneal solute transport rate (PSTR) are age, diabetes, comorbidity, peritonitis, chronic inflammation and frequent use of bio-incompatible PD fluid containing high glucose and glucose degradation products (GDP). Interleukin-6 (IL-6), vascular endothelial growth factor (VEGF), nitric oxide(NO), cancer antigen 125 (CA125) and transforming growth factor-β (TGF-β) have been associated with PSTR. The role of the genetic polymorphism of the above molecules is under investigation.

* E-mail: khoh@snu.ac.kr

We have seen remarkable technical advances in the prevention of peritonitis by allowing less chance of contamination during PD fluid exchange (connectology), along with the development of diagnosis and management protocols. Automated PD facilitating fluid exchange during sleep provides improved quality of life for the patients. Continuous flow PD (CFPD) through potential application of sorbents is also under intensive research.

However, long-term PD is associated with progressive loss of UF capacity, resulting in ultimate discontinuation of PD. This is related to the inflammation, new vessel formation (neoangiogenesis) and fibrotic thickening of the peritoneal membrane (PM). Bio-incompatible PD fluid, along with peritonitis, is the major contributor to the PM change. IL-6, VEGF, TGF-β, connective tissue growth factor (CTGF) are suspected as mediators of the PM injury. There has been recent development of newer biocompatible fluids characterized by neutral pH, non-glucose or low GDP content. Further research will follow in order to develop a more biocompatible PD fluid.

1. Introduction

As of 2006, over 500,000 people in the United States are treated with renal replacement therapies because they have lost the function of their own kidneys (http://www.usrds.org/adr.htm).

Since first application of peritoneal irrigation in a patient suffering from an acute renal failure(ARF) [1], peritoneal dialysis (PD) has been increasingly used as one of the major renal replacement therapies for end-stage renal disease (ESRD) patients. Since continuous ambulatory peritoneal dialysis (CAPD), the most popular mode of PD world wide, was introduced more than thirty years ago, PD is utilized by approximately 120,000 patients on the globe.

2. Basic Principles of Peritoneal Dialysis: Anatomy, Physiology, PET, Kt/V

Uremia is a state of accumulation of various uremic toxins in the blood of patients who suffer from renal failure. Uremic toxins include small molecules like urea, creatinine, electrolytes and large molecules such as β2-microglobin. Protein-bound uremic toxins such as *p*-cresol and ADMA are also known.

Peritoneal dialysis involves transport of solutes and water through the peritoneal membrane. The peritoneum is a serous membrane composed of thin layers of connective tissue covered by a sheet of mesothelium. The peritoneum covers the surface of the intra-abdominal viscera such as stomach, small and large intestines and liver (visceral peritoneum). It also lines the inner surface of the abdominal wall (parietal peritoneum). Actually, there is no membrane called "peritoneal membrane" in the human body. Peritoneal membrane is not an actual membrane but an arbitray nomenclature simplistically meaning the structure composed of the thin mesothelial layer and the connective tissue layers beneath it. It separates two fluid-containing compartments – blood in the peritoneal microcirculation and the PD fluid in the peritoneal cavity. (Figure 1)

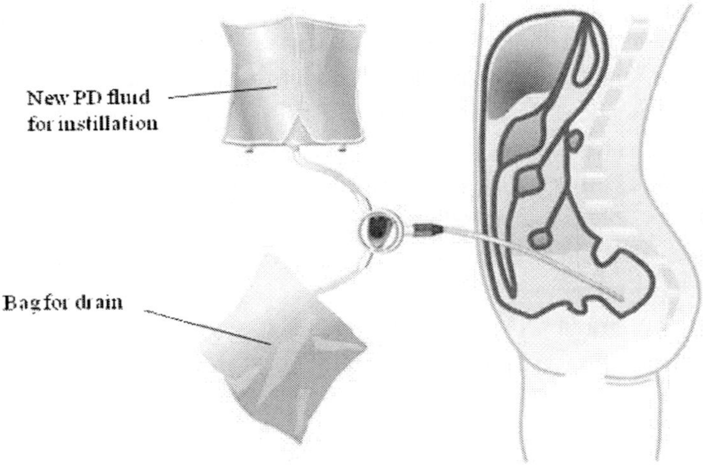

Fig 1. Diagram of the peritoneal cavity and the peritoneal dialysis system. Peritoneal dialysis catheter is inserted into the peritoneal cavity through the anterior abdominal wall. The catheter is a port through which PD fluid is infused and drained. (Courtesy from Fresenius Medical Care).

Blood in the peritoneal capillaries contains high concentrations of uremic solutes and the dialysis fluid in the peritoneal cavity contains sodium, chloride, lactate or bicarbonate and supranormal level of glucose. During a dwell with peritoneal dialysis fluid, three transport processes occur simultaneously- diffusion, convection and ultrafiltration.

1. Functional Structure of the Peritoneum

Peritoneal surface area for a human adult is estimated to be between 1 and 2 m^2 and it approximates the body surface area. The visceral peritoneum, which lines the gut, stomach and other intra-abdominal organs, accounts for about 80% of the total peritoneal surface area. The parietal peritoneum lines the inner surface of the abdominal wall and the diaphragm.

The peritoneal membrane consists of several layers – mesothelium, submesothelial basement membrane, dense interstitial area (compact zone), loose interstitial layer and capillary endothelial layer (Figure 2). Mesothelium is a continuous single cell layer (monolayer) composed of flat mesothelial cells. Luminal surface of the mesothial cell has numerous cytoplasmic extensions called microvilli [2]. Submesothelial basement membrane is a hyaline, homogenous continuous layer lying under the mesothelial layer of visceral, parietal and diaphragmatic peritoneum [3]. Interstitial area is composed of fibroblast and collagen fibers embedded in a gel-like substance.

2. Physiology of Peritoneal Solute Transport and Water Removal

Peritoneal dialysis is a process of solute and water movement between the capillary lumen and peritoneal cavity. Simplistically, peritoneal membrane can be thought of as a semipermeable membrane, through which various substances diffuse down a concentration gradient. Uremic solutes and electrolytes diffuse from the peritoneal capillary into the PD fluid. Glucose and lactate or bicarbonate, which are abundant in the PD fluid, diffuse into the peritoneal capillary. The velocity of diffusion is inversely related with molecular weight of the solute. Urea (MW 60) diffuses more quickly than creatinine (MW 113) or albumin (MW 70,000). Besides, some solute is removed by convection, in which a solute is carried by forced movement of fluid (ultrafiltration). Ultrafiltration is a forced movement of water across the peritoneal membrane. This occurs as a consequence of osmotic gradient driven by high osmolality of PD fluid. PD fluid usually contains supranormal concentrations of glucose (1.36%, 2.27% or 3.86%, respectively). Osmotic gradient is maximal at the beginning of a peritoneal dialysis dwell but is gradually lost over time due to dilution of PD fluid by ultrafiltrate and diffusion of glucose across the peritoneal membrane into the blood.

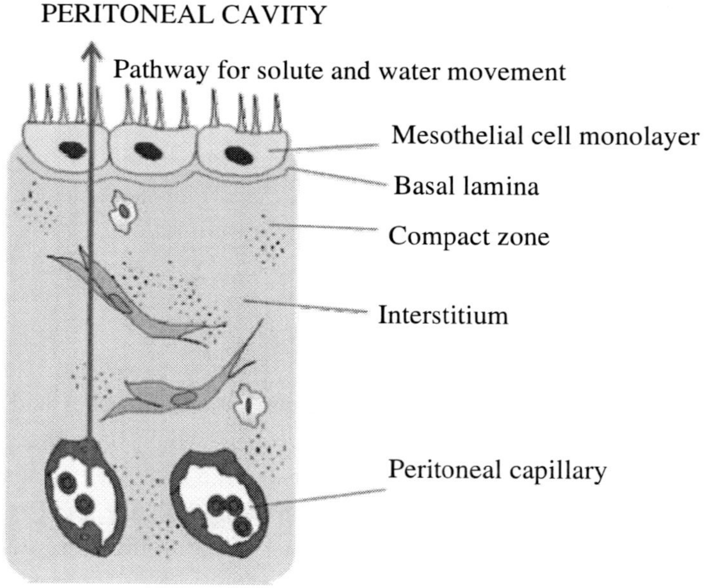

Fig 2. Structure of the normal peritoneal tissue. The peritoneal membrane consists of several layers – mesothelium, submesothelial basement membrane, dense interstitial (compact zone), loose interstitial layer and the capillary endothelium.

Three-pore model is a theory that explains how solutes of varying size move through the peritoneal membrane [4, 5]. In PD, the peritoneum can be regarded as a porous membrane with various pores in three different sizes. Smallest pores (ultrapores) with a diameter < 0.5 nm only permit the passage of water. Small pores (<4nm in diameter) permit water and small solutes to diffuse. Large pores (>15nm in diameter), which correspond to a large cleft in the endothelium, allow the diffusion of macromolecules such as albumin. (Figure 3.)

3. Assessment of the Peritoneal Solute and Water Transport

The speed of the solute and water transport across the peritoneal membrane varies considerably from person to person depending on the effective peritoneal surface area and the intrinsic peritoneal permeability. Peritoneal equilibration test (PET) is a functional test frequently employed in the clinical practice to assess the solute transport and water movement of an individual patient. Peritoneal solute transport is easily assessed by the equilibration ratios between dialysate and plasma for creatinine (D/P cr). For PET, after an overnight dwell, PD fluid is drained out and a new PD fluid in 2.27% glucose bag is infused into the peritoneal cavity and allowed to dwell for 4 hours. Dialysate samples are taken at 0, 2, and 4 hours and plasma sample at 2 hours. The PET results are expressed as the ratio of dialysate creatinine at 4 hours to plasma creatinine at 2 hours (D/P cr); and as the ratio of dialysate glucose at 4 hours to dialysate glucose at time zero (D/D0 glu). Net fluid removal or the difference between infused and drained volume is also recorded.

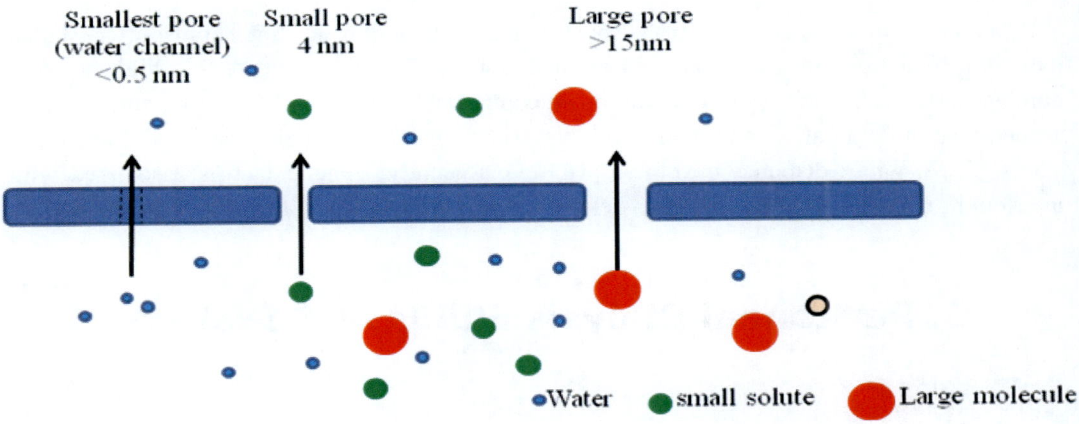

Fig 3. Three pore model explains the movement of solutes and water through the peritoneal membrane.

The higher the dialysate to plasma ratio for creatinine (D/P cr) at 4 hours, the faster the rate of transport of small solutes across the peritoneal membrane. The higher D/Pcr, the lower D/D0 glu. Transport types are classified into four different types depending on the D/Pcr and D/D0 glu ; fast (or high), fast(or high) average, slow(or low) average and slow (or low) transporters. High (fast) transporters absorb glucose rapidly from the PD fluid into the blood. Therefore, high (fast) transporters cannot maintain osmotic gradient in a long dwell which is necessary for net positive fluid removal. (Figure 4.)

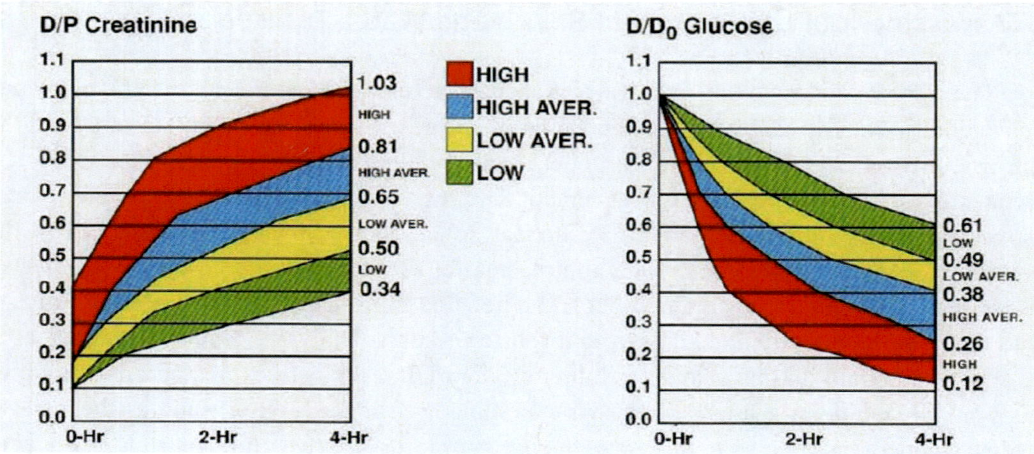

Fig 4. Peritoneal solute transport types are classified into four different groups depending on the PET results (Twardowski et al, Perit Dial Bull 1977).

Numerous factors have been suspected as contributing to high transporter status, including hypoalbuminemia, comorbid disease, duration of PD, exposure to a high glucose, number and severity of peritonitis, and bio-incompatible PD fluid [6-8]. Some authors have argued that inflammation and comorbid disease contribute to high peritoneal transporter status [8, 9], while disputed by others [10, 11]. Recently, genetic factors associated with interleukin-6 have also been known as determining peritoneal solute transport rate [12, 13].

3. Peritoneal Dialysis Fluids and Systems

1. PD Fluids

Three components of PD fluids are electrolyte, buffer, and osmotic agents. For electrolytes, all PD fluids contain sodium, calcium, magnesium, chloride in varying concentrations. For buffering system, PD fluids usually contain lactate for stabilizing pH. Lactate is absorbed into the blood and metabolized in the liver into bicarbonate. Recent technical advances have enabled to manufacture newer PD fluids which contain either bicarbonate alone or mixture of bicarbonate and lactate as the source of buffer. Such newer PD fluids are packed with different solution components in a two- or three-chamber bag, which are mixed immediately before instillation. Bicarbonate should be separated from calcium or magnesium until just before use. Bicarbonate-based solutions have neutral pH and, theoretically, are regarded as more biocompatible than lactate-based solutions with acidic pH. (Table 1) (Figure 5)

Table 1. Components of commercially available PD fluids

	3.86% glucose (conventional)	Icodextrin	Amino acid based	Low GDP (Balance) 3.86% glucose	Low GDP (Physioneal) 3.86% glucose
Lactate (mmol/L)	35	40	40	40	15
Bicarbonate (mmol/L)	-	-	-	-	25
Osmolality (mOsm/kg)	486	285	365	486	483
pH	5.5	5.8	6.7	7.2-7.4	7.2
3-DG (mmol/L)	525	44	-	40	253

3-DG : 3-deoxyglucosone

A

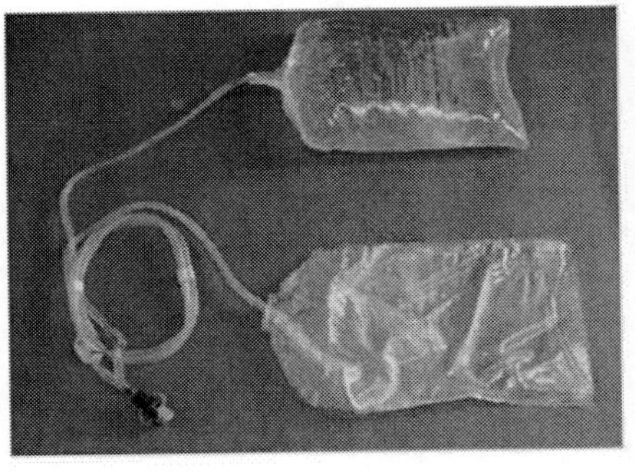

B

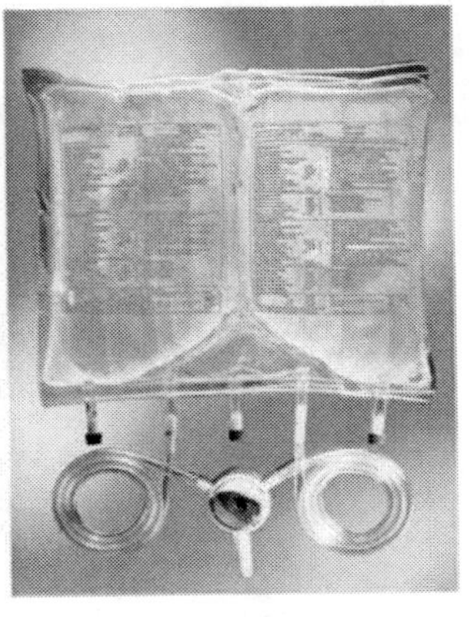

Fig 5. (A) One-chamber and (B) multi-chamber bag systems of PD fluid.

Dextrose (glucose monohydrate, MW 198) is the most commonly used osmotic agent in CAPD solutions. Three different concentrations for dextrose are available among PD fluids – which are 1.5%, 2.5% and 4.3%, respectively. Their true anhydrous glucose (MW 180) concentrations are 1.36%, 2.27% and 3.86%, respectively. The major advantages of dextrose as the osmotic agents lie in inexpensive price and relative safety. However, supranormal concentrations of glucose predisposes the patients into hyperglycemia, hyperlipidemia and obesity since glucose instilled into the peritoneal cavity is absorbed into the systemic circulation and metabolized. Besides, heat sterilization of glucose-containing PD fluid leads to the caramelization of glucose and generates glucose degradation products (GDPs), which are believed to damage the peritoneal membrane (discussed later). Recent technical advances have enabled to reduce the formation of GDP generated during the manufacturing process. That is, the fluid is divided into two or three separate chambers - one chamber containing concentrated glucose in a strong acidic pH and the other containing electrolytes/buffer. When high concentration of glucose is heat-sterilized in a low pH, it generates much less GDP [14-16]. The two or three compartments are mixed just before use.

Alternative osmotic agents have recently been introduced commercially. Icodextrin is a glucose polymer with molecular weight of 20,000. Unlike glucose, the glucose polymer is not absorbed into the peritoneal blood across small pores and, therefore, induces net fluid removal by colloid osmotic pressure. (Figure 6) It does not elevate the blood glucose and promote sustained ultrafiltration in a long dwell [17, 18]. Another product recently developed to reduce glucose-related toxicity is amino acid-based fluid. It was shown in cell culture systems and in animal studies that the administration of amino acid-based is more biocompatible than glucose-based fluids in terms of mesothelial cell viability, ultrastructure, peritoneal immune function and fibrosis [19, 20].

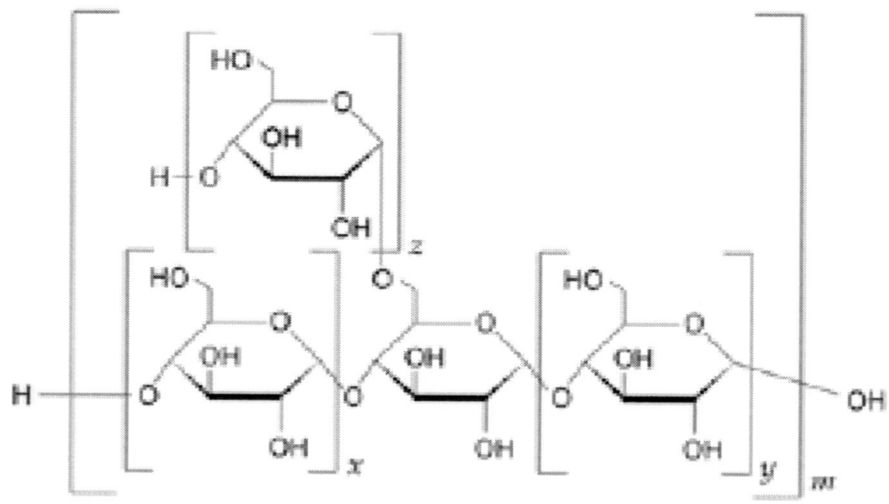

Fig 6. Structure of icodexrtrin. Icodextrin is a glucose polymer with molecular weight of 20,000. Unlike glucose, the glucose polymer is not absorbed into the peritoneal circulation across small pores and, therefore, induces net fluid removal by colloid osmotic pressure.

2. Peritoneal Dialysis Access

Access to the peritoneal cavity is obtained via indwelling catheter implanted through the anterior abdominal wall. The catheter is a port through which PD fluid is infused and drained. The peritoneal catheters are made of silicone rubber or polyurethane and have many side holes along the intraperitoneal portion. (Figure 7) They usually have two Dacron (polyester) cuffs which provoke local inflammation and fibrosis. This fibrous tissue surrounding the peritoneal catheter fixes the catheter in the abdominal wall and prevents migration of bacteria from outside. The most typical catheters are straight or curled Tenckhoff catheters but alternate catheters have been devised in order to prevent the catheter migration or outflow obstruction.

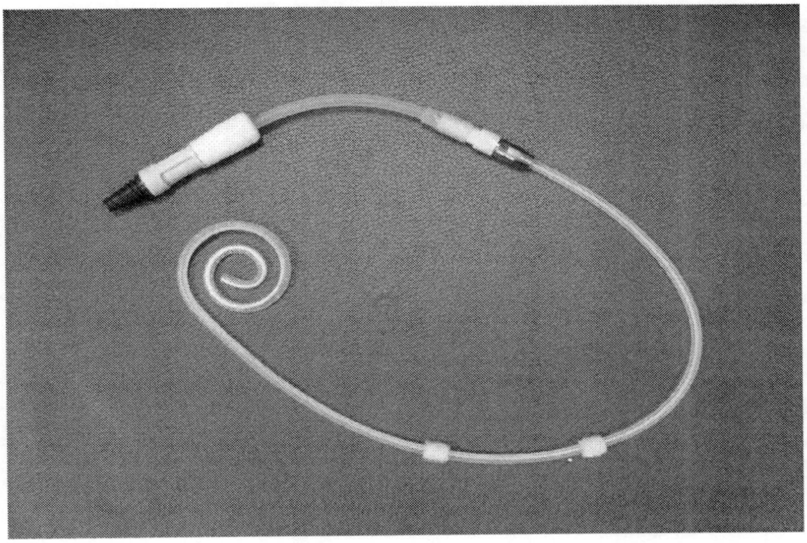

Fig 7. Tenckhoff peritoneal catheter and transfer set. Tenckhoff PD catheter has two Dacron (polyester) cuffs which help fix the catheter to the subcutaneous tunnel of the abdominal wall and prevents migration of bacteria from outside.

4. Mode of Peritoneal Dialysis

1. Continuous Ambulatory Peritoneal Dialysis (CAPD)

CAPD is the most common mode of dialysis in the world. In CAPD, the peritoneal fluid is constantly present in the peritoneal cavity around the clock. The patient exchanges PD fluid manually three to five times a day. The patient drains spent dialysate first, flushes the tubing and finally instills new PD fluid into the peritoneal cavity. Each manual exchange usually takes between 20 and 30 minutes.

2. Automated Peritoneal Dialysis (APD)

APD is a new dialysis method that utilizes a machine called cycler. Instead of timed manual exchange of PD fluids, cycler drains and refills the peritoneal cavity automatically and programmably while the patient is asleep. It is a rapidly growing method and, in some countries including the United States, more patients are placed on APD than CAPD. Depending on the presence or absence of PD fluids in the peritoneal cavity during daytime, APD is further divided into continuous cycler-assisted PD (CCPD) and nocturnal PD (NPD). In CCPD, a patient, on top of nocturnal automated fluid exchange, carries PD fluid in the abdomen throughout the daytime, although no exchange of PD fluid is performed during the daytime. In NPD, the cycler fully drains out the abdomen at the end of nocturnal automated exchange. In this case, the patient spends the daytime with no fluid in the abdomen. (Figure 8)

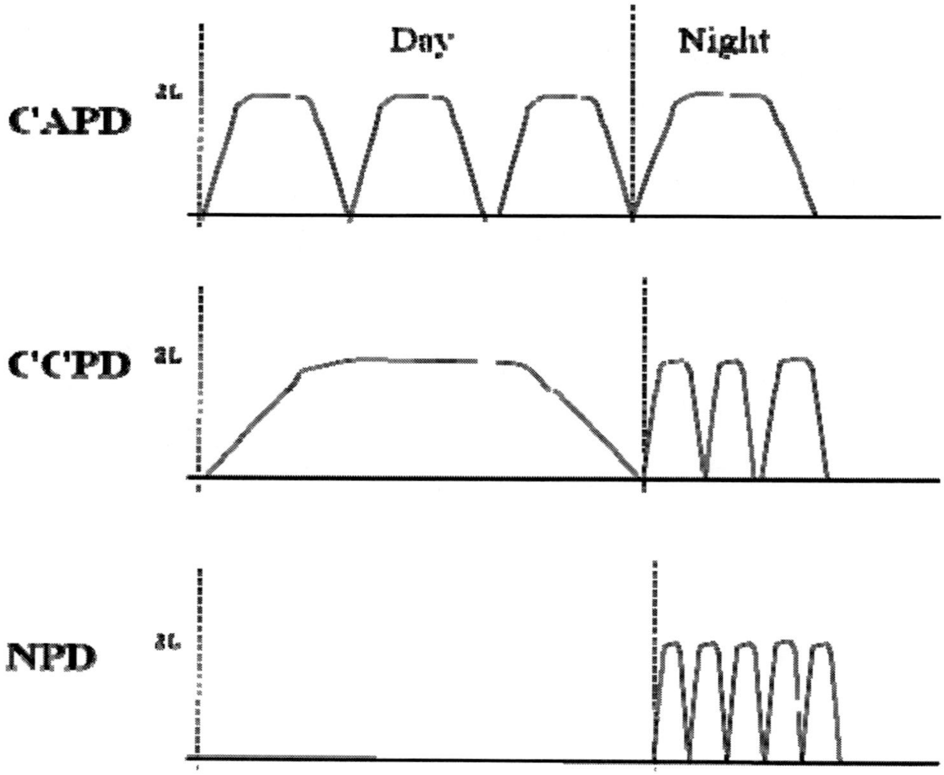

Fig 8. Various modes of peritoneal dialysis. CAPD: continuous ambulatory peritoneal dialysis, CCPD : continuous cycler-assisted peritoneal dialysis, NPD : nocturnal peritoneal dialysis

5. Clinical Issues in Peritoneal Dialysis

1. Peritonitis

Peritonitis is an inflammatory condition of the peritoneum induced by various invading microorganisms such as bacteria, fungi and mycobacteria. Peritonitis remains the Achilles heel of PD. The typical symptoms and signs of peritonitis are abdominal pain, turbid effluent, nausea, vomiting and diarrhea. In clinical practice, the incidence of peritonitis ranges from one episode in every 18 to 36 months. However, recent advances of PD fluid connection system (connectology) has dramatically reduced the chance of contamination during PD solution exchange and, hence, the total incidence of peritonitis. When peritonitis develops, intraperitoneal administration of antibiotics or anti-fungal agents is usually effective in eradicating the pathogen. However, some peritonitis cases are refractory despite immediate and adequate treatment and eventually lead to peritoneal catheter removal, discontinuation of peritoneal dialysis and/or patient death. Repeated episodes of peritonitis may lead to the thickening and fibrosis of the peritoneum and, eventually, discontinuation of PD (discussed later).

2. Adequacy

The volume of peritoneal dialysis fluid and the frequency of bag exchange should be prescribed in order to ensure adequate removal of solute from uremic patients. The adequate removal of solute can be monitored in various ways, the most representative of which are measuring the clearance of creatinine (CrCl) and urea (Kt/Vurea) by urea kinetic modeling. Kt/Vurea is a ratio of total weekly urea clearance (Kt) divided by the urea distribution volume (V). V is equal to the total body water and is proportional to the body weight. The consensus target for Kt/V in peritoneal dialysis is now 1.7.

3. UF Failure and Volume Overload

Patients with advanced renal insufficiency who cannot excrete water and solutes through the urine typically accumulate sodium and water in their body. Therefore, they develop hypertension (high blood pressure) and edema (swelling of the legs and other parts of body), both of which culminate in cardiovascular events. For the balance of sodium and water, both the input and output of sodium should be controlled. For the input, sodium restriction is encouraged to the patients. For the output, doctors prescribe various PD fluids depending on the fluid status of a patient. For dextrose-based PD solutions, the higher the concentration of glucose in the PD fluid, the larger ultrafiltration volume the patient usually achieves. Icodextrin, a large carbohydrate polymer that is not absorbed across the peritoneal membrane, enables a long-term maintenance of osmotic gradient in the peritoneal cavity and, thus, is suitable for long nocturnal dwell.

Some patients who do not achieve UF volume of more than 400 mL after 4 hour dwell with 4.25% dextrose PD solution are in a state of ultrafiltration failure. High transporters in whom glucose diffuses rapidly from the peritoneal cavity into the systemic circulation are in a risk of developing UF failure (type I UF failure). Other causes for UF failure are also known.

Development of UF failure has been attributed to the peritoneal new vessel formation, thickening and fibrosis which result from long-term instillation of bio-incompatible PD fluid with supranormal glucose level and high GDP content. Recurrent peritonitis has also been suspected as damaging the peritoneal membrane, ultimately resulting in UF failure.

4. Toxicity of Glucose and Glucose Degradation Products

Glucose has been most widely used as an osmotic agent for PD fluids. It is relatively safe, inexpensive, osmotically effective and easily metabolized into H_2O and CO_2 in our body. However, long-term exposure of the peritoneal membrane to the very high concentrations of glucose brings about several adverse effects both locally and systemically.

It was shown that glucose in high concentrations has direct adverse effects on the mesothelial cell functions. High glucose induces alterations in complement synthesis and up-regulations of inflammatory cytokines such as monocyte chemoattractant protein-1 (MCP-1)

[21-23] and transforming growth factor –β (TGF-β) [21, 24]. High glucose has been shown to induce the phenotypic change of mesothelial cells from epithelial cell type into a mesenchymal phenotype that is ready to synthesize fibrotic molecules in a process called epithelial-to-mesenchymal transition (EMT) [25, 26]. This process is important in developing peritoneal fibrosis in response to high glucose. Mechanisms of glucose toxicity is mediated by the polyol, protein kinase C (PKC) and hexosamine pathways. High glucose has been shown to be detrimental to other cell types, as well, including adipocytes, leukocytes, fibroblasts and peritoneal vascular endothelial cells.

Glucose degradation products (GDPs) are low molecular weight compounds that are produced during breakdown of glucose. GDPs are formed while glucose-based PD fluids are heat-sterilized during manufacture or during prolonged storage in room temperature. Various GDPs such as acetaldehyde, formaldehyde, glyoxal, methylglyoxal, 3-deoxyglucosone (3-DG), 3,4-dideoxyglucosone-3-ene(3,4-DGE) have been identified from glucose-based PD fluid. GDPs affect mesothelial cell proliferation and viability [27, 28]. Exposure of human peritoneal mesothelial cells to GDPs results in a pro-inflammatory response – up-regulation of vascular cell adhesion molecule-1 (VCAM-1), interleukin-6, and interleukin-8. Methylglyoxal, one of the GDPs in the PD fluid, enhances the release of vascular endothelial growth factor (VEGF) in mesothelial and endothelial cells [29]. VEGF increases new vessel formation in the peritoneum and renders the peritoneal capillaries to be hyper-permeable to large molecules.

In addition to the direct toxicity of high glucose and GDPs, glucose-based dialysis fluids are associated with accumulation of advanced glycation end products (AGEs) in the peritoneal membrane. Both glucose and GDPs are strong inducers of AGE [30]. AGEs are formed when glucose or reactive carbonyl compounds (RCOs) such as GDPs combine with amino groups in the side chains of proteins without the help of enzymes (nonenzymatically). AGEs cross-link matrix molecules such as collagen and injure the structural integrity of proteins. Recently, it has been shown that AGEs exert their harmful effect via receptor for AGE (RAGE) [31]. RAGE is expressed in the peritoneum and inflammatory cells. AGE-RAGE interaction induces multiple signaling pathways, leading to secretion of inflammatory cytokines, adhesion molecules and production of growth factors such as TGF-β and VEGF [32]. (Figure 9).

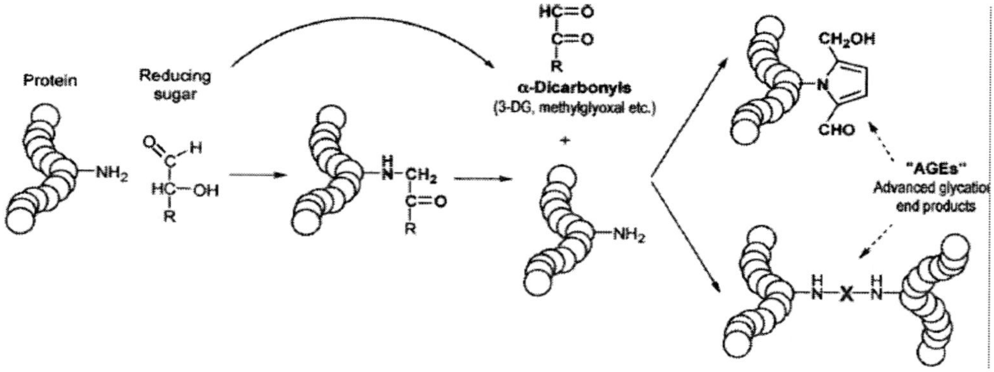

Fig 9. GDP and AGE formation. (Brownlee et al, N Eng J Med 1988)

6. Issues in Long-term Peritoneal Dialysis

1. Biocompatibility

Lactate based low pH PD fluid with glucose as the main osmotic agent has been used for a long time since peritoneal dialysis was conceived. It is still the most commonly used PDF in the world. However, it has been recently recognized that the conventional glucose-based PD fluid with acidic pH and GDPs has many bio-incompatibility issues, as mentioned above. Conventional PDF has been demonstrated in vitro and in animal studies to increase the production of inflammatory cytokines, VEGF, and TGF-β [24, 33]. It finally leads to peritoneal fibrosis and encapsulating peritoneal sclerosis (discussed later). Besides, glucose absorbed from the PD fluid increases the blood glucose concentration in diabetic patients and leads to obesity and metabolic disturbances.

Scientists have been developing more biocompatible PD fluids, neither glucose-based, nor GDP-containing and with neutral pH. Glucose-based PDFs with low GDP content typically have multi-chamber system, separating glucose from buffer and electrolytes. Less GDP is produced during heat sterilization of the multi-chamber PD fluid. There are two different types of non-glucose containing PDF commercially available these days. Amino acid containing PDF contains 1.1% amino acid. It was originally designed to supplement amino acid to malnourished PD patients. It could be considered as more biocompatible than conventional PDF, as it does not contain glucose and GDPs. Icodextrin, a glucose polymer, is a large molecule derived from starch. It has been used as an alternative osmotic agent in a long overnight dwell in CAPD or a long daytime dwell in APD. It has normal osmolality, absence of glucose and low GDP content. It has better biocompatibility than conventional PDF. However, more than one bags per day for amino acid based PDF or icodextrin-based PDF is not recommended because excessive amino acid or icodextrin use might aggravate metabolic acidosis or hypermaltosemia (a state of high maltose in the blood). Research should be warranted for a more biocompatible osmotic agent which can replace glucose more perfectly in every PD exchange.

2. Encapsulating Peritoneal Sclerosis

Encapsulating peritoneal sclerosis (EPS) is one of the most serious complications in the peritoneal dialysis. It is characterized by marked peritoneal thickening and fibrosis, resulting in bowel obstruction and death. Although the pathogenesis of EPS has not been elucidated, risk factors for developing EPS have been known. Long-term PD therapy has been suggested as a major risk factor. A survey in Japan reported incidence of 0.7% at 5 years of PD treatment but the incidence goes up to 5.9% at 10 years of PD [34]. Histologic changes of the peritoneum associated with prolonged PD, exposure to bio-incompatible PD fluid and recurrent peritonitis are postulated to be causally related. Acidity, high osmolality, high levels of GDP and high glucose concentration in the conventional PD fluid are known to be toxic to the mesothelium and other components of the peritoneum. It is necessary to investigate whether newer biocompatible PD fluids recently introduced into clinical practice might reduce the incidence of EPS in the future.

7. Future Prospects

1. Clinical benefit of new generation fluids

Newer biocompatible solutions recently introduced into clinical practice have been demonstrated to be better than conventional PDF in terms of peritoneal cell and inflammatory markers. It looks promising for better preservation of peritoneal membrane function and prevention from EPS. Some researchers suggested a beneficial effect of low GDP fluid in terms of preserving residual renal function [35] However, clinical benefit of these new generation fluids has yet to be proved in the future by well-designed clinical trials with larger scale and sufficient follow-up period.

2. Search for an Alternative Osmotic Agent and a New PD Solution

New generation PD fluid based on amino acid or icodextrin as the osmotic agent has some limitations as discussed above. Efforts should be exerted for developing alternative osmotic agent that can completely replace glucose with much better biocompatibility and long-term safety [36-38].

3. Peritoneal Membrane Preservation

Various agents that can prevent or treat peritoneal membrane degeneration or EPS should be sought for. Researchers are investigating the efficacy and safety of GDP scavengers that can prevent formation of AGEs and crosslink breakers that can remove preformed AGEs. Various agents interfering with intracellular pathways mediating glucose-mediated cytotoxicity – aldose reductase inhibitors, protein kinase C pathway inhibitors – are also being evaluated. Additives to PD fluid such as antioxidants, low molecular weight heparin, hyaluronan and indomethacin are actively investigated. Agents targeting the growth factors and cytokines such as transforming growth factor-β (TGF-β)[39], hepatocyte growth factor (HGF), connective tissue growth factor (CTGF) that are involved in the peritoneal inflammation and fibrosis [40] are also promising. Gene therapy using anti-angiogenic and anti-fibrotic genes might protect the peritoneal membrane and salvage the deteriorating membrane [41]. Reconstituting the denuded and inflamed peritoneum with mesothelial or bone marrow-derived stem cells is another promising field of research in the future.

4. Technical Advances in Dialysis Machines

Automated peritoneal dialysis (APD) is the fastest growing dialysis technique in the world. The rapid development in this field has enabled the development of new technology. It also facilitates varying prescription and delivery of dialysis customized to the individual patient.

For patients treated by APD, a larger dose of dialysis are generally prescribed. On-line preparation of PD fluid by mixing water with appropriate electrolyte and osmolytes could be a new solution to the high cost and practical problems in transporting, storing and handling large volumes. However, on-line preparation of PD fluid is limited to a few technical reports yet and remains to be investigated in the future.

Continuous flow PD (CFPD) is a current state-of-the-art [42-43]. It relies on a 2-3 L dwell volume and continuous dialysate flow rate at 100-300 mL/min. A high flow rate in CFPD needs to be backed up by a dual lumen catheter or two separate catheters. It also necessitates a technical support to generate or regenerate large volumes of sterile PD fluid. CFPD can ensure sufficient solute clearance, especially for large, anuric (with no urine production) patients or high transporters who do not acquire enough ultrafiltration volume during CAPD. However, technical challenges remain in terms of catheter design, ultrafiltration control and real time measurement for intraperitoneal volume.

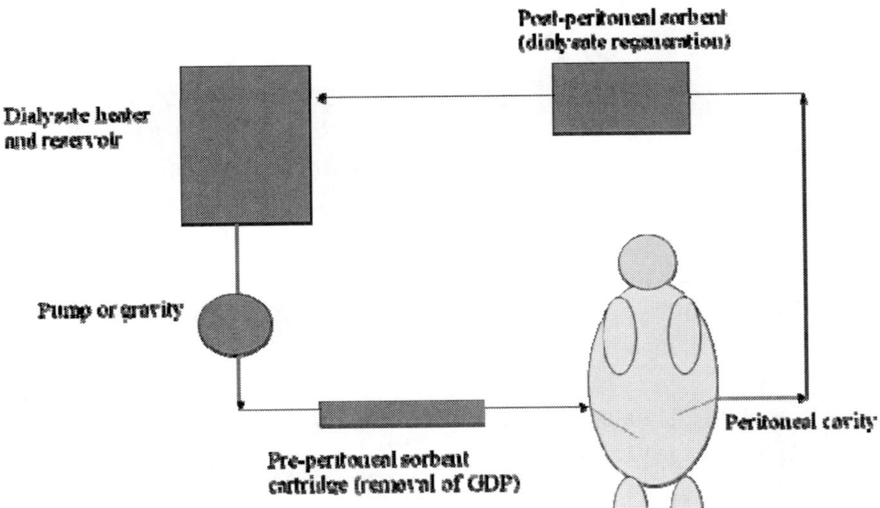

Fig 10. Schema of sorbent assisted peritoneal dialysis (modified from Winchester et al. Contrib Nephrol 2006)

5. Sorbents in PD

Uremic toxins which are protein-bound include p-cresol, homocysteine, and asymmetric dimethylarginine (ADMA). These molecules are hardly removed by dialysis but may be amenable to sorbent removal. Middle molecules and low molecular weight proteins including β2-microglobin, AGEs, leptin and proinflammatory cytokines and chemokines are also uremic toxins that are poorly removed by conventional dialysis modalities. Sorbents have the potential for an effective removal of these uremic toxins. Sorbents can be applied to the CFPD system and assist the regeneration of PD fluid. (Figure 10)

Conclusion

Peritoneal dialysis is a well established dialysis method world wide. Basically, it is a home-based therapy and provides independence from hospital schedules. It is a slow, continuous therapy and, therefore, brings about less hemodynamic stress and is also suited for patients with cardiovascular instability. Technical development has seen advances in the new biocompatible PD fluid and automated machines that can be customized to the patient's medical condition and social needs. Incidence of peritonitis, which has been a crucial problem in the clinical practice of PD, has decreased dramatically along with the development in connectology. However, issues of biocompatibility and glucose-mediated toxicity in association with long-term preservation of the peritoneal membrane has yet to be solved. Challenges lie in the field of new PD fluid development and therapeutic interventions for peritoneal membrane deterioration, EPS and adequate delivery of PD.

References

[1] Fine J, Frank H, Seligman A. The treatment of acute renal failure by peritoneal irrigation. *Ann. Surg.* 1946; 124: 857.

[2] Odor DL. Observations of the rat mesothelium with the electron and phase microscopes. *Am. J. Anat.* 1954; 95 (3): 433.

[3] Baron MA. Structuree of the intestinal peritoneum in man. Am J Anat 1941; 69: 439.

[4] Flessner MF. Peritoneal transport physiology: insights from basic research. *J. Am. Soc. Nephro*l. 1991; 2 (2): 122.

[5] Rippe B, Stelin G, Haraldsson B. *Computer simulations of peritoneal fluid transport in CAPD.* Kidney Int 1991; 40 (2): 315.

[6] Margetts PJ, McMullin JP, Rabbat CG, Churchill DN. Peritoneal membrane transport and hypoalbuminemia: cause or effect? *Perit. Dial. Int.* 2000; 20 (1): 14.

[7] Chung SH, Heimburger O, Stenvinkel P, Bergstrom J, Lindholm B. Association between inflammation and changes in residual renal function and peritoneal transport rate during the first year of dialysis. *Nephrol. Dial Transplant* 2001; 16 (11): 2240.

[8] Davies SJ, Phillips L, Naish PF, Russell GI. Quantifying comorbidity in peritoneal dialysis patients and its relationship to other predictors of survival. *Nephrol. Dial Transplant* 2002; 17 (6): 1085.

[9] Chung SH, Chu WS, Lee HA, et al. Peritoneal transport characteristics, comorbid diseases and survival in CAPD patients. *Perit Dial Int* 2000; 20 (5): 541.

[10] Oh KH, Moon JY, Oh J, et al. Baseline peritoneal solute transport rate is not associated with markers of systemic inflammation or comorbidity in incident Korean peritoneal dialysis patients. *Nephrol. Dial Transplant* 2008; 23 (7): 2356.

[11] Rodrigues AS, Almeida M, Fonseca I, et al. Peritoneal fast transport in incident peritoneal dialysis patients is not consistently associated with systemic inflammation. *Nephrol. Dial Transplant* 2006; 21 (3): 763.

[12] Gillerot G, Goffin E, Michel C, et al. Genetic and clinical factors influence the baseline permeability of the peritoneal membrane. *Kidney Int* 2005; 67 (6): 2477.

[13] Hwang Y-H, Son M-J, Yang J, et al. Effects of interleukin-6 T15A single nucleotide polymorphism on baseline peritoneal solute transport rate in incident peritoneal dialysis patients. *Perit. Dial Int* 2009; 29 (1).

[14] Wieslander AP, Kjellstrand PT, Rippe B. Heat sterilization of glucose-containing fluids for peritoneal dialysis: biological consequences of chemical alterations. *Perit. Dial. Int* 1995; 15 (7 Suppl): S52.

[15] Ledebo I, Wieslander A, Kjellstrand P. Can we prevent the degradation of glucose in peritoneal dialysis solutions? *Perit. Dial Int* 2000; 20 Suppl 2: S48.

[16] Kjellstrand P, Martinson E, Wieslander A, Holmquist B. Development of toxic degradation products during heat sterilization of glucose-containing fluids for peritoneal dialysis: influence of time and temperature. *Perit. Dial Int* 1995; 15 (1): 26.

[17] Posthuma N, ter Wee PM, Verbrugh HA, et al. Icodextrin instead of glucose during the daytime dwell in CCPD increases ultrafiltration and 24-h dialysate creatinine clearance. *Nephrol. Dial. Transplant* 1997; 12 (3): 550.

[18] Mistry CD, Gokal R, Peers E. A randomized multicenter clinical trial comparing isosmolar icodextrin with hyperosmolar glucose solutions in CAPD. MIDAS Study Group. Multicenter Investigation of Icodextrin in Ambulatory Peritoneal Dialysis. *Kidney Int* 1994; 46 (2): 496.

[19] Chan TM, Leung JK, Sun Y, Lai KN, Tsang RC, Yung S. Different effects of amino acid-based and glucose-based dialysate from peritoneal dialysis patients on mesothelial cell ultrastructure and function. *Nephrol. Dial Transplant* 2003; 18 (6): 1086.

[20] Zareie M, van Lambalgen AA, ter Wee PM, et al. Better preservation of the peritoneum in rats exposed to amino acid-based peritoneal dialysis fluid. *Perit. Dial Int* 2005; 25 (1): 58.

[21] Wong TY, Phillips AO, Witowski J, Topley N. Glucose-mediated induction of TGF-beta 1 and MCP-1 in mesothelial cells in vitro is osmolality and polyol pathway dependent. *Kidney Int* 2003; 63 (4): 1404.

[22] Lee SK, Kim BS, Yang WS, Kim SB, Park SK, Park JS. High glucose induces MCP-1 expression partly via tyrosine kinase-AP-1 pathway in peritoneal mesothelial cells. *Kidney Int* 2001; 60 (1): 55.

[23] Haslinger B, Mandl-Weber S, Sellmayer A, Lederer SR, Sitter T. Effect of high glucose concentration on the synthesis of monocyte chemoattractant protein-1 in human peritoneal mesothelial cells: involvement of protein kinase C. *Nephron* 2001; 87 (4): 346.

[24] Wang T, Chen YG, Ye RG, Li SL, Li HQ, Chen YX. Effect of glucose on TGF-beta 1 expression in peritoneal mesothelial cells. *Adv. Perit. Dial.* 1995; 11: 7.

[25] Ito T, Yorioka N, Yamamoto M, Kataoka K, Yamakido M. Effect of glucose on intercellular junctions of cultured human peritoneal mesothelial cells. *J. Am. Soc. Nephrol.* 2000; 11 (11): 1969.

[26] Medcalf JF, Walls J, Pawluczyk IZ, Harris KP. Effects of glucose dialysate on extracellular matrix production by human peritoneal mesothelial cells (HPMC): the role of TGF-beta. *Nephrol. Dial Transplant* 2001; 16 (9): 1885.

[27] Witowski J, Korybalska K, Wisniewska J, et al. Effect of glucose degradation products on human peritoneal mesothelial cell function. *J. Am. Soc. Nephrol.* 2000; 11 (4): 729.

[28] Witowski J, Bender TO, Gahl GM, Frei U, Jorres A. Glucose degradation products and peritoneal membrane function. *Perit. Dial. Int.* 2001; 21 (2): 201.

[29] Inagi R, Miyata T, Yamamoto T, et al. Glucose degradation product methylglyoxal enhances the production of vascular endothelial growth factor in peritoneal cells: role in the functional and morphological alterations of peritoneal membranes in peritoneal dialysis. *FEBS Lett* 1999; 463 (3): 260.

[30] Welten AG, Schalkwijk CG, ter Wee PM, Meijer S, van den Born J, Beelen RJ. Single exposure of mesothelial cells to glucose degradation products (GDPs) yields early advanced glycation end-products (AGEs) and a proinflammatory response. *Perit. Dial. Int.* 2003; 23 (3): 213.

[31] Yan SF, Ramasamy R, Naka Y, Schmidt AM. Glycation, inflammation, and RAGE: a scaffold for the macrovascular complications of diabetes and beyond. *Circ. Res.* 2003; 93 (12): 1159.

[32] Nakamura S, Tachikawa T, Tobita K, et al. Role of advanced glycation end products and growth factors in peritoneal dysfunction in CAPD patients. *Am. J. Kidney Dis.* 2003; 41 (3 Suppl 1): S61.

[33] Zareie M, Hekking LH, Welten AG, et al. Contribution of lactate buffer, glucose and glucose degradation products to peritoneal injury in vivo. *Nephrol. Dial Transplant* 2003; 18 (12): 2629.

[34] Kawanishi H, Kawaguchi Y, Fukui H, et al. Encapsulating peritoneal sclerosis in Japan: a prospective, controlled, multicenter study. *Am. J. Kidney Dis.* 2004; 44 (4): 729.

[35] Kim S, Oh J, Chung W, Ahn C, Kim SG, Oh KH. Benefits of biocompatible PD fluid for preservation of residual renal function in incident CAPD patients: a 1-year study. Nephrol Dial Transplant 2009 in press, doi:10.1093/ndt/gfp054, Epub 2009 Mar 03

[36] Smit W, de Waart DR, Struijk DG, Krediet RT. Peritoneal transport characteristics with glycerol-based dialysate in peritoneal dialysis. *Perit. Dial. Int.* 2000; 20 (5): 557.

[37] Van Biesen W, Boer W, De Greve B, et al. A randomized clinical trial with a 0.6% amino acid/ 1.4% glycerol peritoneal dialysis solution. *Perit. Dial. Int.* 2004; 24 (3): 222.

[38] Van Biesen W, Vanholder R, Lameire N. Recent developments in osmotic agents for peritoneal dialysis. *Adv. Ren. Replace Ther.* 1998; 5 (3): 218.

[39] Margetts PJ, Oh KH, Kolb M. Transforming growth factor-beta: importance in long-term peritoneal membrane changes. *Perit. Dial. Int.* 2005; 25 Suppl 3: S15.

[40] Oh KH, Margetts PJ. Cytokines and growth factors involved in peritoneal fibrosis of peritoneal dialysis patients. *Int. J. Artif Organs* 2005; 28 (2): 129.

[41] Margetts PJ, Gyorffy S, Kolb M, et al. Antiangiogenic and antifibrotic gene therapy in a chronic infusion model of peritoneal dialysis in rats. *J. Am. Soc. Nephrol.* 2002; 13 (3): 721.

[42] Dell'Aquila R, Rodighiero MP, Spanó E, Di Loreto P, et al. Advances in the technology of automated, tidal, and continuous flow peritoneal dialysis. Perit Dial Int. 2007;27 Suppl 2:S130-7.

[43] Amerling R, Glezerman I, Savransky E, Dubrow A, Ronco C. Continuous flow peritoneal dialysis: principles and applications. Semin Dial. 2003;16(4):335-40.

In: Nephrology – Dialysis - Transplantation
Editors: Endre Kruger and Kelemen Hahn

ISBN 978-1-60741-736-1
© 2009 Nova Science Publishers, Inc.

Chapter IV

Role of Plasminogen Activator Inhibitor-1 in the Development of Renal Interstitial Fibrosis

Takashi Oda*
Department of Nephrology,
National Defense Medical College, Saitama, Japan

Abstract

Because renal interstitial fibrosis occurs in virtually all the progressive renal diseases leading to end-stage renal failure controlling it would be a reasonable therapeutic strategy. Plasminogen activator inhibitor-1 (PAI-1) is the main regulator of plasminogen activator-plasmin system and is attracting attention as one of the key molecules in the development of renal fibrosis. It is weakly expressed in normal kidney, but its expression is upregulated in various renal diseases leading to renal fibrosis. We have shown in mice with unilateral ureteral obstruction, a model for progressive renal interstitial fibrosis, that genetically engineered mice deficient for PAI-1 develop less renal fibrosis than wild-type mice. We have also shown in spontaneously hypercholesterolemic rat, a model of chronic progressive renal disease with massive proteinuria, that drugs reported to inhibit PAI-1 *in vitro*, such as angiotensin II type-1 receptor blocker and peroxisome proliferator-activated receptor gamma (PPAR-γ) agonist, inhibit renal PAI-1 expression and have a significant renoprotective effect. PAI-1 is therefore a promising therapeutic target for chronic progressive renal disease.

This chapter describes the evidence for the important role of PAI-1 and the value of therapeutic approaches targeting PAI-1 in progressive renal fibrosis.

---

* Address correspondence to: Takashi Oda, M.D., Department of Nephrology, National Defense Medical College, 3-2 Namiki, Tokorozawa-shi, Saitama 359-8513, Japan. Phone: +81-4-2995-1609; Fax: +81-4-2996-5201; E-mail: takashio@ndmc.ac.jp

Introduction

The number of end-stage renal disease (ESRD) patients that require dialysis or renal transplant is increasing world-wide, imposing enormous medical and socioeconomic burdens [1]. The importance of renal disease as the public health problems has been widely recognized in accordance with the understanding of chronic kidney disease (CKD) as the major independent risk factor of cardiovascular disease and ESRD [2]. The initial causes of damage and the progression mechanisms may differ between different renal diseases, but renal interstitial fibrosis is part of the final common pathway to ESRD [3-5]. Controlling it would thus be a reasonable therapeutic strategy for the prevention or arrest of progressive renal disease. Renal interstitial fibrosis is a consequence of perturbation of the normal balance between the synthesis and degradation of extracellular matrix (ECM), and two intrarenal protease cascades—the matrix metalloproteinase (MMP) cascade and the plasminogen activator (PA)/plasmin cascade—are thought to act in concert in the degradation process [6, 7]. Plasmin appears to play a pivotal role in regulating these cascades because both most MMPs and PAs are secreted in the form of inactive proenzymes whose conversion to active enzymes requires plasmin action. Blockade of plasmin generation would thus repress the activities of both plasmin and MMPs, whereas tissue inhibitors of metalloproteinases (TIMPs) would not affect plasmin activity [6]. Plasminogen activator inhibitor-1 (PAI-1), a regulator of the PA/plasmin cascade, is a powerful fibrosis-promoting molecule and has therefore recently been attracting attention as a promising therapeutic target [8-10]. PAI-1 expression is almost undetectable in normal kidneys, but is upregulated in various renal diseases leading to renal fibrosis [11-15]. We showed that genetically engineered mice deficient for PAI-1 develop less renal fibrosis than wild-type mice in response to unilateral ureteral obstruction (UUO) [16]—which produces a model of progressive interstitial fibrosis. Krag *et al.* [17] reported that PAI-1 deficiency attenuates the glomerular and interstitial ECM deposition observed in mice overexpressing transforming growth factor-β (TGF-β), and Matsuo *et al.* [18] have demonstrated that overexpression of PAI-1 aggravates the interstitial fibrosis in mice with UUO. Although it has been widely accepted that PAI-1 plays a significant role in renal fibrosis whether its profibrotic effect is due to its regulatory function in the PA/plasmin cascade is still controversial because PAI-1 has many effects—such as those on cell adhesion, detachment, and migration—that are independent of the PA/plasmin cascade [8, 19, 20].

This review summarizes our data as well as recently reported findings regarding the role of PAI-1 in renal fibrosis and summarizes therapeutic strategies targeting PAI-1 in progressive renal disease.

Overview of PA/Plasmin System and PAI-1

The PA/plasmin system is best known for its role in blood fibrinolysis. The system is initiated by conversion of the plasma zymogens plasminogen to the active protease plasmin by a physiological activator, either urokinase-type plasminogen activator (uPA) or tissue-type plasminogen activator (tPA). Besides regulating the blood fibrinolysis, plasmin has been shown to exert a broad range of functions by degrading substrates other than fibrin. Plasmin can itself degrade ECM proteins such as fibronectin or laminin and can proteolytically activate pro-MMPs and latent growth factors (such as TGF-β and basic FGF), thereby contributing to cell migration, embryogenesis, wound healing, angiogenesis, and tumor growth and dissemination [7, 21]. The conversion of plasminogen to plasmin is tightly regulated by the PA inhibitors (PAIs) PAI-1, PAI-2, PAI-3 (also called as protein C inhibitor), protease nexin 1, and neuroserpin [20, 22]. PAI-1 has been investigated extensively because it the primary physiological inhibitor of both tPA and uPA *in vivo*. It is a single-chain glycoprotein with a molecular weight of 50 kDa and is a member of the SERPIN (for SERine Protease INhibitor) family. The PAI-1 gene has been reported to have its expression increased by variety of factors such as tumor necrosis factor-α, TGF-β [23], interleukin-1, endotoxin (lipopolysaccharide) [24], vascular endothelial growth factor-β [25], glucocorticoids [26], renin [27], and angiotensin [28] and has been regarded as a kind of acute phase response gene. Although the primary sources of PAI-1 in normal and pathological conditions are still controversial, many cell types have been shown to produce PAI-1: endothelial cells, smooth muscle cells, fibroblasts, renal tubular epithelial cells, and mesangial cells [8, 10]. PAI-1 is rapidly secreted in an active form after synthesis and is not stored within cells, although platelets store a latent form of PAI-1 and secrete it upon cellular activation. The conversion of the latent form to the active form is reportedly due to a conformational change in the reactive center loop of the inhibitor [29]. Active PAI-1 forms irreversible 1:1 molar complexes with active PAs, which are subsequently endocytozed and degraded. Thus, PAI-1 is thought to reduce ECM degradation by inhibiting plasmin generation and MMP activation (pro-MMPs are activated by plasmin and by activated MT1-MMP induced by uPA, both of which are inhibited by PAI-1 [30, 31]). A PAI-1-induced decrease in fibrinolysis is thought to result in fibrin deposition in target organs, subsequently leading to the infiltration of cells such as fibroblasts and macrophages that induce ECM deposition. These mechanisms, *i.e.* reduction of ECM degradation and induction of fibrin deposition and subsequent cell infiltration, are thought to be the mechanisms responsible for profibrotic effect of PAI-1 that are dependent on its regulatory role in PA/plasmin cascade.

PAI-1 also has effects that are independent of PA/plasmin cascade. It modulates the behavior of several cells and plays an important role in inflammation, wound healing, angiogenesis, and tumor metastasis [19, 20]. The molecular details of these effects are not clear, but one of the known important pathways is a complex interplay among PAI-1, vitronectin, uPAR [32], and integrin receptors [8, 20]. Both integrins and uPAR can bind to vitronectin, and their binding is competitively inhibited by PAI-1. The binding site of both uPAR and PAI-1 has been shown to be the somatomedin B domain on the NH_2 terminus of vitronectin, and this site is immediately adjacent to the only RGD sequence site in vitronectin that binds to integrins. Thus, PAI-1 binds to vitronectin and prevents it from attaching to cells by blocking integrin and/or uPAR binding sites [33]. PAI-1 is also reported to modulate cell migration by binding to cell surface-bound uPA. PA-1 binds to uPAR-bound uPA on the cell surface and induces the internalization of resulting uPAR-uPA-PAI-1 complex, thereby inhibiting uPA-induced cell migration. The interactions of the above factors are very complex, and conflicting observations that PAI-1 can either inhibit or promote cell migration have been reported. This may be due to the differences in the cell type, the local concentration of PAI-1, and the presence or absence of vitronectin, uPA, and uPAR. Furthermore, PAI-1 has been shown to be a chemoattractant molecule that induces migration of certain type of cells independent of its interactions with uPA, tPA, or vitronectin. This function is induced by the binding of PAI-1 to low-density lipoprotein receptor-related protein (LRP) on the cell surface and subsequent activation of the Jac/Stat signaling pathway [34]. In keeping with this concept, we showed PAI-1 itself attracts monocytes *in vitro* [16]. Although the reported effects of PAI-1 on cell behavior *in vitro* are sometimes conflicting as described above, its effect on cells *in vivo* is almost always promigratory [16, 35, 36]. This promigratory action of PAI-1 contributes to tissue fibrosis by causing the accumulation of profibrotic cells, such as macrophages and myofibroblasts.

Renal Fibrosis and PAI-1

PAI-1 is scarcely detected in normal kidney, but it's expression has been reported to be up-regulated in various human and experimental renal diseases leading to renal fibrosis, such as focal segmental glomerulosclerosis [37], diabetic nephropathy [38], allograft nephropathy [13], hypertensive nephropathy [39], obstructive nephropathy [16], protein-overload proteinuria [40], radiation nephropathy [41], aging [15], anti-Thy-1 nephritis [42], lupus nephritis [43], cyclosporine-induced glomerulosclerosis [14], crescentic anti-glomerular basement membrane glomerulonephritis [44], and so on. This suggests that PAI-1 plays a role in the development of renal fibrosis, and to find out whether its increased expression is the cause or the consequence of renal inflammation and fibrosis, we investigated the renal response to injury in mice genetically deficient in PAI-1.

In wild-type (+/+) mice, PAI-1 is prominently induced by UUO, a model of acute and aggressive renal interstitial fibrosis, to a degree corresponding to the progression of renal fibrosis (Figure 1A), but in PAI-1-deficient mice (-/-) the renal interstitial fibrosis is significantly attenuated (Figure 1B) [16]. Unexpectedly, we found no significant difference between PAI-1 -/- mice and +/+ mice in terms of the intrarenal PA activity or plasmin activity associated with UUO. On the other hand, the recruitment of interstitial monocytes/macrophages and myofibroblasts (Figure 2) was significantly reduced in -/- mice as compared with +/+ mice. Because these cells have been reported to be implicated in the fibrogenic process by producing fibrogenic cytokines that induce ECM production, the blunting of inflammatory response may account for the antifibrotic effects of PAI-1 deficiency. Northern blotting for TGF-β and collagens I and III showed the expression of these fibrogenic molecules to be more pronounced in UUO kidneys from +/+ mice than in those from -/- mice, which is consistent with PAI-1 deficiency blunting the inflammatory response. A similar protective effect of PAI-1 deficiency was found in the chronic and milder interstitial fibrosis induced by protein-overload proteinuria [45]. These data were impressive in light of evidence that the deficiency of another protease inhibitor also prominently upregulated in association with interstitial fibrosis, TIMP-1, had no protective effect on UUO kidneys [46]. Furthermore, Matsuo *et al.* [18] recently supported our findings by showing that the interstitial fibrosis with increased macrophage infiltration in UUO kidneys from mice overexpressing PAI-1 is worse than that in UUO kidneys from wild-type mice.

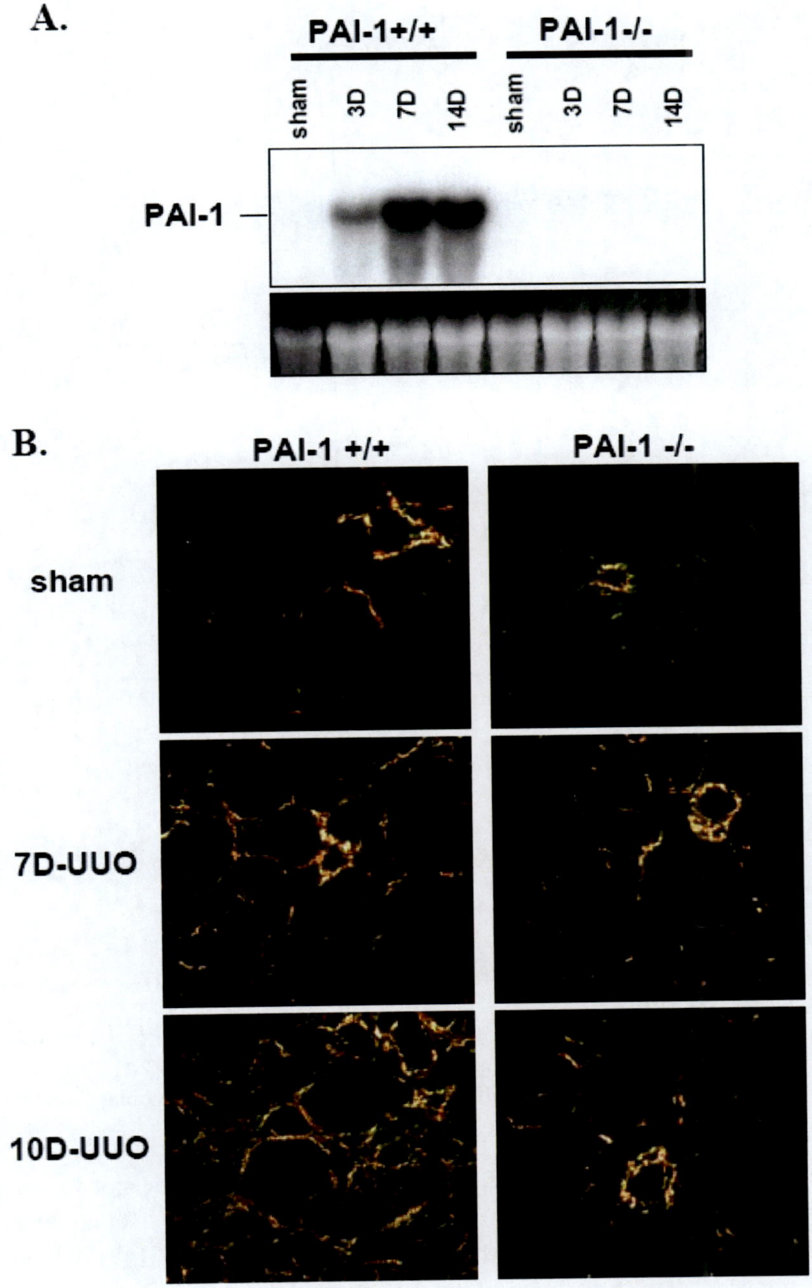

Figure 1. (A) Representative Northern blotting of renal mRNA levels for PAI-1 in the kidneys of sham-operated PAI-1 +/+ and PAI-1 -/- mice and the kidneys of PAI-1 +/+ and PAI-1 -/- mice 3, 7, and 14 days (D) after UUO operation. Prominent PAI-1 induction is evident in the +/+ UUO mice. (B) Representative photomicrographs of Sirius red staining in kidneys of sham-operated PAI-1 +/+ and PAI-1 -/- mice and kidneys of UUO PAI-1 +/+ and PAI-1 -/- mice 7 and 14 D after the UUO operation. The Sirius red-stained interstitial area is smaller in the PAI-1 -/- mice. Reprinted from reference (16) with permission.

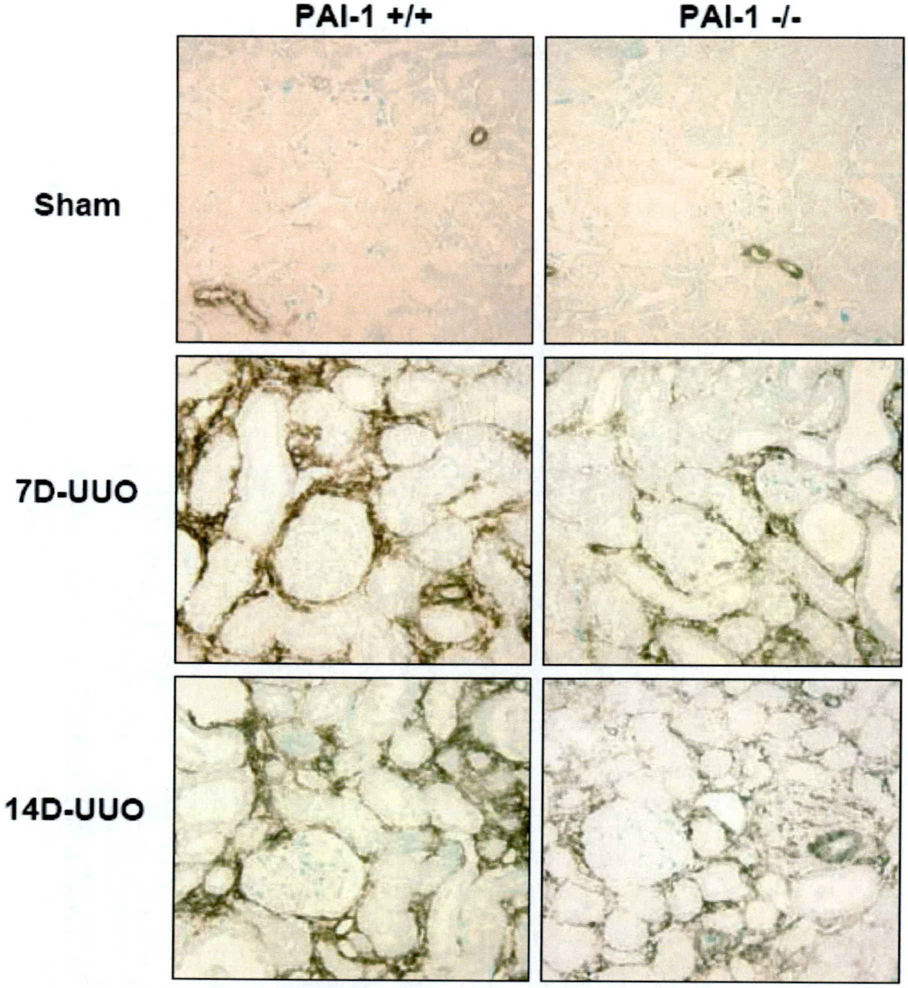

Figure 2. Representative photomicrographs of immunoperoxidase staining for α-smooth muscle actin-positive interstitial myofibroblasts in the kidneys of sham-operated and UUO PAI-1 +/+ and PAI-1 -/- mice 7 and 14 days (D) after the UUO operation. Renal infiltration of myofibloblasts was decreased by PAI-1 deficiency. Reprinted from reference (16) with permission.

These results suggest that the profibrotic effect of PAI-1 is due not to the regulatory function of PAI-1 in the PA/plasmin cascade but to the ability of PAI-1 to modulate receptor-dependent cell behavior. In keeping with this concept, Edgtton *et al.* (47) demonstrated that plasmin did not show any protective effect on interstitial fibrosis in UUO kidneys. They found the interstitial fibrosis in the UUO kidney of plasminogen -/- mice, which are totally plasmin deficient, to be less severe than that in the UUO kidney of plasminogen +/+ mice. Indeed, in the UUO kidney of normal mice, despite the progressive increase of PAI-1 protein and PAI activity with the progression of interstitial fibrosis, plasmin activity was abruptly increased after UUO surgery as assessed by casein gel zymography [48] (Figure 3A) and *in situ* zymography [49] (Figure 3B).

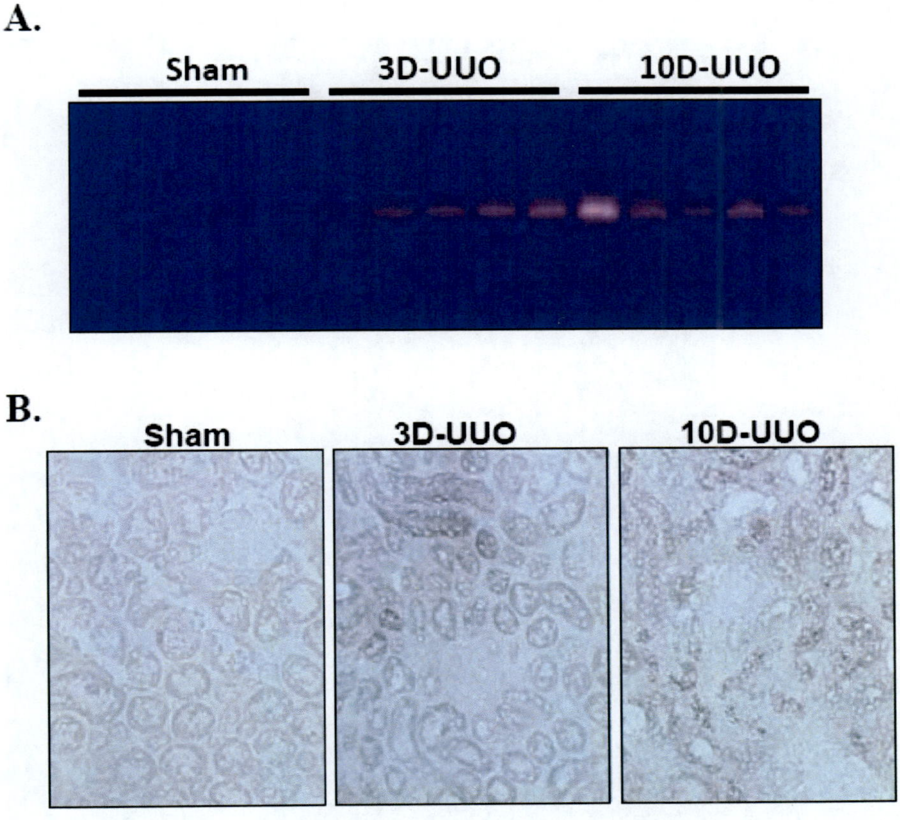

Figure 3. (A) Representative casein gel zymography results for plasmin activities in proteins isolated from sham-operated mice and UUO mice 3 and 10 days (D) after the UUO operation. (B) Representative photomicrographs of *in situ* zymography results for plasmin activity in kidneys of sham-operated mice and UUO mice 3 and 10 D after the UUO operation. Both assays showed plasmin activities to be increased by UUO.

The interstitial infiltration of macrophages and myofibroblasts, in contrast, correlated positively with the degree of renal fibrosis in the UUO kidney (Figure 4). Thus, the progression of fibrosis in the UUO kidney correlated well with the increased PAI-1 expression and the infiltration of macrophages or myofibroblasts but did not correlate with the decrease in plasmin activity (Oda *et al.* manuscript in preparation).

Most of the reports of investigations of the effects of genetic PAI-1 modulation in renal disease models other than those produced by UUO or protein overload are consistent with a renoprotective effect of PAI-1 deficiency. Nicholas *et al.* [50] used the mouse model of streptozotocin-induced diabetes and reported that the albuminuria and fibronectin levels in PAI-1 -/- mice were lower than those in wild-type mice. They attributed this effect to the ability of PAI-1 to regulate TGF-β expression by binding to uPAR and activating the ERK/MAPK pathway. In the db/db mouse model, too, the PAI-1 -/- genotype was associated with reduced albuminuria and renal collagen levels, but there it was also associated with a higher mortality rate [51]. PAI-1 -/- also attenuated the kidney disease induced by genetic overexpression of TGF-β, decreasing both glomerular and interstitial ECM deposition [17].

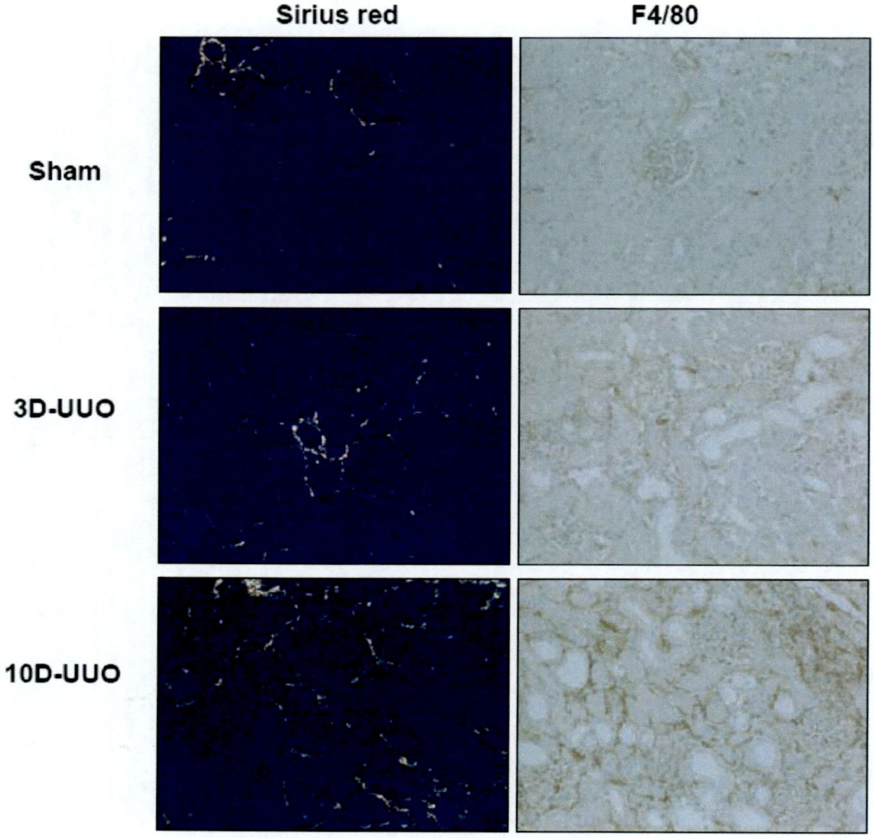

Figure 4. Representative photomicrographs of Sirius red staining and immunoperoxidase staining for F4/80-positive interstitial macrophages in kidneys of sham-operated mice and UUO mice 3 and 10 days (D) after the UUO operation. Interstitial macrophage infiltration correlated well with interstitial fibrosis level.

Here again, this attenuation was not associated with the change in protease activity but was associated with ECM synthesis. In the anti-glomerular basement membrane (GBM) crescentic glomerulonephritis model, PAI-1-/- mice showed fewer glomerular crescents, less glomerular fibrin deposition, less leukocyte infiltration, and less collagen accumulation than did wild-type mice. In contrast, PAI-1 ++/++ mice showed increased glomerular crescent formation, more glomerular fibrin deposition, increased leukocyte infiltration, and extensive collagen accumulation [44]. A different outcome was reported in a passive model of anti-GBM glomerulonephritis [52], where the renal injury in the PAI-1 -/- mice was far more severe than that in the wild-type mice, the PAI-1 -/- mice showed much higher activation of TGF-β than did +/+ mice, and systemic neutralization of TGF-β significantly attenuated the severity of the injury in the PAI-1 -/- mice. It was therefore thought that PAI-1 deficiency increased the activities of renal uPA and tPA (again, plasmin levels did not differ between -/- and +/+ mice), activating latent TGF-β and thereby exacerbating the renal damage.

Like TIMP-1, PAI-1 may also have beneficial effects under certain pathological conditions, especially in vascular remodeling after intimal injury or in chronic transplant arteriopathy [10].

PAI-1 deficiency has also been reported to protect against tissue fibrosis in other organs, although the suggested mechanism of its antifibrotic effect differs in each report. Wang *et al.* [53] reported that PAI-1 deficiency reduces hepatic fibrosis after bile duct obstruction mainly by increasing tPA activity and thereby activating hepatocyte growth factor. They found a significant increase in tPA activity in PAI-1-/- mice but found no difference between PAI-1 -/- and +/+ mice in terms of uPA or plasmin activities. Eitzman *et al.* [54] reported that the pulmonary fibrosis induced by bleomycin was significantly milder in PAI-1-/- mice than in +/+ mice and was significantly worse in ++/++ mice than in +/+ mice. They suggested that these effects of PAI-1 reflected increased pulmonary fibrin deposition and subsequent cell infiltration resulting from decreased fibrinolysis due to downregulated plasmin generation. Hattori *et al.* [55], however, showed that increased fibrin clearance could not account for the antifibrotic effects of PAI-1 deficiency in this model because bleomycin-induced pulmonary fibrosis is not attenuated by a genetic deficiency of fibrinogen.

Thus, the net effects of PAI-1 on tissue fibrosis are essentially similar in liver, lung, and kidney but the mechanism of action in each organ is controversial.

Therapeutic Strategy for Progressive Renal Disease That Modulates PAI-1 Expression

Above facts suggest that inhibiting renal PAI-1 expression can be a potential pharmacological strategies for chronic progressive renal disease.

A unique therapeutic approach targeting PAI-1 has been extensively analyzed by Huang and co-workers [56-58]. They inhibited PAI-1 by using a dominant-negative mutant of human PAI-1 (PAI-1R) that binds vitronectin normally but does not inhibit PAs. Both in anti-Thy-1 nephritis and db/db mice, intravenous or intraperitoneal injection of mutant PAI-1R caused significant increases in glomerular plasmin generation, reductions in proteinuria, and decreases in glomerular ECM deposition. PAI-1R thus reduces glomerulosclerosis by competing with endogenous PAI-1 thereby restoring plasmin generation and increasing plasmin-dependent degradation of ECM.

Renin and angiotensin induce PAI-1 expression, and inhibitors of the renin-angiotensin system (RAS)—*i.e.* angiotensin converting enzyme (ACE) inhibitors and angiotensin type-1 receptor blockers (ARBs)—inhibit the expression of PAI-1. There is much recent evidence that RAS inhibitors have significant protective effects on CKD, and the inhibitory effect on PAI-1 is thought to contribute to this renoprotective effect of RAS inhibitors [15, 59]. Some CKD patients treated with RAS inhibitors nonetheless experience end-stage renal failure, and some CKD patients cannot use medications inhibiting the RAS because their blood pressure is low or their serum potassium concentration is high. Because there is thus a need for alternative therapeutic strategies and because peroxisome proliferator-activated receptor gamma (PPAR-γ) agonists have been reported to inhibit PAI-1 *in vitro* and *in vivo* (60-62), we investigated the effect of PPAR-γ agonists on CKD. We first analyzed the effect of the PPAR-γ agonist pioglitazone on spontaneously hypercholesterolemic (SHC) rats, a model of chronic progressive renal disease with massive proteinuria, and found that long-term (6 months) treatment with it inhibited the renal PAI-1 expression and macrophage infiltration and exerted a significant renoprotective effect similar to that of the ARB candesartan [63]. Generally, plasmin is expected to decrease with the upregulation of PAI-1 because PAI-1 inhibits PAs and thereby inhibits plasmin generation. We found in our study, however, that PAI-1 and plasmin activity increased concomitant with the progression of renal fibrosis and that both PAI-1 and plasmin activity decreased with the regression of fibrosis in response to treatments with either pioglitazone or candesartan (Figure 5), indicating that the profibrotic action of PAI-1 is not due to inhibition of plasmin activity. Interestingly, pioglitazone also reduced the urinary protein excretion more than candesartan did. Benigni *et al.* [64] also reported that pioglitazone significantly reduced proteinuria and had a renoprotective effect in passive Heymann nephritis. They proposed that the antiproteinuric effect of pioglitazone is due to transcriptional upregulation of the nephrin gene in podocytes. A PPAR-γ agonist has also been reported to protect podocytes from damage in progressive glomerulosclerosis with urinary protein [65].

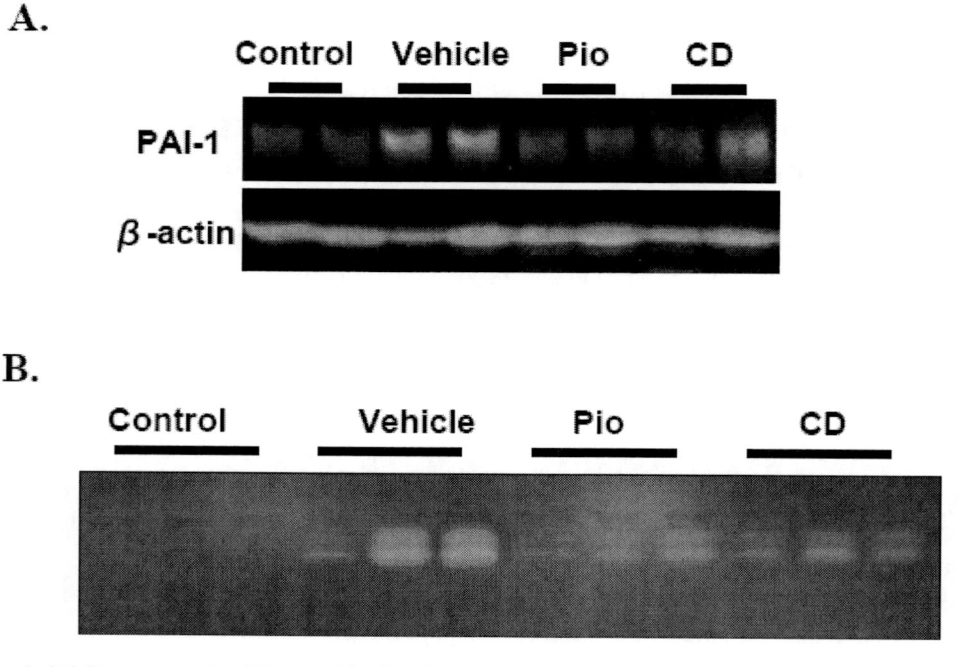

Figure 5. (A) Representative Western blotting for renal PAI-1 and β-actin in control rats and in SHC rats treated with vehicle, pioglitazone (Pio), or candesartan (CD). (B) Representative casein gel zymography results for plasmin activities in proteins isolated from control rats and from SHC rats treated with vehicle, Pio, or CD. Levels of PAI-1 and plasmin activity increased concomitantly after disease development and were decreased by treatments with Pio or CD. Reprinted from reference (63) with permission.

We then investigated the effects of a RAS inhibitor and a PPAR-γ agonist and their combination on the UUO kidney, a model of progressive interstitial fibrosis without proteinuria, so that we could evaluate the renoprotective effect of a PPAR-γ agonist independent of urine protein reduction and evaluate the additive effect of a PPAR-γ agonist and RAS-inhibitor (Higashi *et al.*, manuscript submitted).

Clinically, the evaluation of this drug combination is important because PPAR-γ agonists are supposed to be used in combination with RAS inhibitors, which are already widely used as the standard medication for most CKD patients. The renal total collagen level was increased prominently by UUO, but this increase was significantly attenuated by treatment with either pioglitazone or candesartan and was further attenuated by treatment with both. Similarly, PAI-1 mRNA and protein levels were prominently increased by UUO, this overexpression was significantly reduced by pioglitazone or candesartan treatment, and combination treatment resulted in further reduction.

The attenuation of interstitial fibrosis and reduction of macrophage infiltration in the renal cortex showed the same trend as the reduction in PAI-1. Combination therapy with pioglitazone and candesartan thus exerts an additive protective effect on renal fibrosis by inhibiting renal PAI-1 expression and this combination could be an effective treatment for CKD.

Conclusion

PAI-1 is involved in the process by which various renal diseases lead to end-stage renal failure. It is multifunctional protein that exerts profibrotic effect, possibly by protease-dependent mechanisms (regulating plasmin generation and MMP-activation) and/or protease-independent mechanisms (interacting with uPAR, vitronectin, or LRP). It is thus a potent fibrosis-promoting molecule and a promising therapeutic target for progressive renal disease. Drugs that inhibit PAI-1 expression, such as RAS inhibitors and PPAR-γ agonists, protect the kidney from fibrosis, and in combination these drugs show additive antifibrotic effects on progressive renal disease.

The mechanism of the profibrotic action of PAI-1 is controversial and should be clarified in the future. This would lead to the development of more specific and effective inhibitors of PAI-1 that would show stronger antifibrotic effects with minimal side effects.

Acknowledgments

We are grateful to our colleague Ms. Yasuko Sugimoto for her expert secretarial assistance and to Dr. Allison A. Eddy, Division of Nephrology, Department of Pediatrics, University of Washington, for valuable advice and discussion and to Ms. Tatsuyo Harasawa, Central Research Laboratory, National Defense Medical College, for excellent technical assistance.

References

[1] Collins, A.J., Foley, R., Herzog, C., Chavers, B., Gilbertson, D., Ishani, A., Kasiske, B., Liu, J., Mau, L.W., McBean, M., et al. 2008. Excerpts from the United States Renal Data System 2007 annual data report. *Am. J. Kidney Dis* 51:S1-320.

[2] Levey, A.S., Atkins, R., Coresh, J., Cohen, E.P., Collins, A.J., Eckardt, K.U., Nahas, M.E., Jaber, B.L., Jadoul, M., Levin, A., et al. 2007. Chronic kidney disease as a global public health problem: approaches and initiatives - a position statement from Kidney Disease Improving Global Outcomes. *Kidney Int.* 72:247-259.

[3] Eddy, A.A. 1996. Molecular insights into renal interstitial fibrosis. *J. Am. Soc. Nephrol.* 7:2495-2508.

[4] Eddy, A.A. 1998. Interstitial fibrosis in hypercholesterolemic rats: role of oxidation, matrix synthesis, and proteolytic cascades. *Kidney Int* 53:1182-1189.

[5] Eddy, A.A., and Neilson, E.G. 2006. Chronic kidney disease progression. *J. Am. Soc. Nephrol.* 17:2964-2966.

[6] Mignatti, P., and Rifkin, D.B. 1993. Biology and biochemistry of proteinases in tumor invasion. *Physiol Rev* 73:161-195.

[7] Vassalli, J.D., Sappino, A.P., and Belin, D. 1991. The plasminogen activator/plasmin system. *J. Clin. Invest* 88:1067-1072.

[8] Eddy, A.A. 2002. Plasminogen activator inhibitor-1 and the kidney. *Am. J. Physiol. Renal Physiol* 283:F209-220.

[9] Eddy, A.A., and Fogo, A.B. 2006. Plasminogen activator inhibitor-1 in chronic kidney disease: evidence and mechanisms of action. *J. Am. Soc. Nephrol.* 17:2999-3012.

[10] Rerolle, J.P., Hertig, A., Nguyen, G., Sraer, J.D., and Rondeau, E.P. 2000. Plasminogen activator inhibitor type 1 is a potential target in renal fibrogenesis. *Kidney Int* 58:1841-1850.

[11] Keeton, M., Eguchi, Y., Sawdey, M., Ahn, C., and Loskutoff, D.J. 1993. Cellular localization of type 1 plasminogen activator inhibitor messenger RNA and protein in murine renal tissue. *Am. J. Pathol.* 142:59-70.

[12] Moll, S., Menoud, P.A., Fulpius, T., Pastore, Y., Takahashi, S., Fossati, L., Vassalli, J.D., Sappino, A.P., Schifferli, J.A., and Izui, S. 1995. Induction of plasminogen activator inhibitor type 1 in murine lupus-like glomerulonephritis. *Kidney Int* 48:1459-1468.

[13] Wang, Y., Pratt, J.R., Hartley, B., Evans, B., Zhang, L., and Sacks, S.H. 1997. Expression of tissue type plasminogen activator and type 1 plasminogen activator inhibitor, and persistent fibrin deposition in chronic renal allograft failure. *Kidney Int.* 52:371-377.

[14] Duymelinck, C., Dauwe, S.E., Nouwen, E.J., De Broe, M.E., and Verpooten, G.A. 1997. Cholesterol feeding accentuates the cyclosporine-induced elevation of renal plasminogen activator inhibitor type 1. *Kidney Int.* 51:1818-1830.

[15] Ma, L.J., Nakamura, S., Whitsitt, J.S., Marcantoni, C., Davidson, J.M., and Fogo, A.B. 2000. Regression of sclerosis in aging by an angiotensin inhibition-induced decrease in PAI-1. *Kidney Int.* 58:2425-2436.

[16] Oda, T., Jung, Y.O., Kim, H.S., Cai, X., Lopez-Guisa, J.M., Ikeda, Y., and Eddy, A.A. 2001. PAI-1 deficiency attenuates the fibrogenic response to ureteral obstruction. *Kidney Int* 60:587-596.

[17] Krag, S., Danielsen, C.C., Carmeliet, P., Nyengaard, J., and Wogensen, L. 2005. Plasminogen activator inhibitor-1 gene deficiency attenuates TGF-beta1-induced kidney disease. *Kidney Int* 68:2651-2666.

[18] Matsuo, S., Lopez-Guisa, J.M., Cai, X., Okamura, D.M., Alpers, C.E., Bumgarner, R.E., Peters, M.A., Zhang, G., and Eddy, A.A. 2005. Multifunctionality of PAI-1 in fibrogenesis: evidence from obstructive nephropathy in PAI-1-overexpressing mice. *Kidney Int* 67:2221-2238.

[19] Lijnen, H.R. 2005. Pleiotropic functions of plasminogen activator inhibitor-1. *J. Thromb Haemost* 3:35-45.

[20] Dellas, C., and Loskutoff, D.J. 2005. Historical analysis of PAI-1 from its discovery to its potential role in cell motility and disease. *Thromb. Haemost* 93:631-640.

[21] Castellino, F.J., and Ploplis, V.A. 2005. Structure and function of the plasminogen/plasmin system. *Thromb Haemost* 93:647-654.

[22] Yepes, M., and Lawrence, D.A. 2004. Neuroserpin: a selective inhibitor of tissue-type plasminogen activator in the central nervous system. *Thromb Haemost* 91:457-464.

[23] Sawdey, M.S., and Loskutoff, D.J. 1991. Regulation of murine type 1 plasminogen activator inhibitor gene expression in vivo. Tissue specificity and induction by lipopolysaccharide, tumor necrosis factor-alpha, and transforming growth factor-beta. *J. Clin. Invest.* 88:1346-1353.

[24] Emeis, J.J., and Kooistra, T. 1986. Interleukin 1 and lipopolysaccharide induce an inhibitor of tissue-type plasminogen activator in vivo and in cultured endothelial cells. *J. Exp. Med.* 163:1260-1266.

[25] Olofsson, B., Korpelainen, E., Pepper, M.S., Mandriota, S.J., Aase, K., Kumar, V., Gunji, Y., Jeltsch, M.M., Shibuya, M., Alitalo, K., et al. 1998. Vascular endothelial growth factor B (VEGF-B) binds to VEGF receptor-1 and regulates plasminogen activator activity in endothelial cells. *Proc. Natl. Acad. Sci. USA* 95:11709-11714.

[26] Medcalf, R.L., Van den Berg, E., and Schleuning, W.D. 1988. Glucocorticoid-modulated gene expression of tissue- and urinary-type plasminogen activator and plasminogen activator inhibitor 1 and 2. *J. Cell Biol* .106:971-978.

[27] Nguyen, G., Delarue, F., Berrou, J., Rondeau, E., and Sraer, J.D. 1996. Specific receptor binding of renin on human mesangial cells in culture increases plasminogen activator inhibitor-1 antigen. *Kidney Int* 50:1897-1903.

[28] Vaughan, D.E., Lazos, S.A., and Tong, K. 1995. Angiotensin II regulates the expression of plasminogen activator inhibitor-1 in cultured endothelial cells. A potential link between the renin-angiotensin system and thrombosis. *J. Clin. Invest* 95:995-1001.

[29] Mottonen, J., Strand, A., Symersky, J., Sweet, R.M., Danley, D.E., Geoghegan, K.F., Gerard, R.D., and Goldsmith, E.J. 1992. Structural basis of latency in plasminogen activator inhibitor-1. *Nature* 355:270-273.

[30] Baricos, W.H., Cortez, S.L., el-Dahr, S.S., and Schnaper, H.W. 1995. ECM degradation by cultured human mesangial cells is mediated by a PA/plasmin/MMP-2 cascade. *Kidney Int* 47:1039-1047.

[31] Kazes, I., Delarue, F., Hagege, J., Bouzhir-Sima, L., Rondeau, E., Sraer, J.D., and Nguyen, G. 1998. Soluble latent membrane-type 1 matrix metalloprotease secreted by human mesangial cells is activated by urokinase. *Kidney Int* 54:1976-1984.

[32] Waltz, D.A., Natkin, L.R., Fujita, R.M., Wei, Y., and Chapman, H.A. 1997. Plasmin and plasminogen activator inhibitor type 1 promote cellular motility by regulating the interaction between the urokinase receptor and vitronectin. *J. Clin. Invest* 100:58-67.

[33] Stefansson, S., and Lawrence, D.A. 1996. The serpin PAI-1 inhibits cell migration by blocking integrin alpha V beta 3 binding to vitronectin. *Nature* 383:441-443.

[34] Degryse, B., Neels, J.G., Czekay, R.P., Aertgeerts, K., Kamikubo, Y., and Loskutoff, D.J. 2004. The low density lipoprotein receptor-related protein is a motogenic receptor for plasminogen activator inhibitor-1. *J. Biol. Chem.* 279:22595-22604.

[35] Pedersen, H., Grondahl-Hansen, J., Francis, D., Osterlind, K., Hansen, H.H., Dano, K., and Brunner, N. 1994. Urokinase and plasminogen activator inhibitor type 1 in pulmonary adenocarcinoma. *Cancer Res* 54:120-123.

[36] Bajou, K., Noel, A., Gerard, R.D., Masson, V., Brunner, N., Holst-Hansen, C., Skobe, M., Fusenig, N.E., Carmeliet, P., Collen, D., et al. 1998. Absence of host plasminogen activator inhibitor 1 prevents cancer invasion and vascularization. *Nat Med* 4:923-928.

[37] Hamano, K., Iwano, M., Akai, Y., Sato, H., Kubo, A., Nishitani, Y., Uyama, H., Yoshida, Y., Miyazaki, M., Shiiki, H., et al. 2002. Expression of glomerular plasminogen activator inhibitor type 1 in glomerulonephritis. *Am. J. Kidney Dis* 39:695-705.

[38] Paueksakon, P., Revelo, M.P., Ma, L.J., Marcantoni, C., and Fogo, A.B. 2002. Microangiopathic injury and augmented PAI-1 in human diabetic nephropathy. *Kidney Int* 61:2142-2148.

[39] Tamaki, K., Okuda, S., Nakayama, M., Yanagida, T., and Fujishima, M. 1996. Transforming growth factor-beta 1 in hypertensive renal injury in Dahl salt-sensitive rats. *J. Am. Soc. Nephrol.* 7:2578-2589.

[40] Eddy, A.A., and Giachelli, C.M. 1995. Renal expression of genes that promote interstitial inflammation and fibrosis in rats with protein-overload proteinuria. *Kidney Int.* 47:1546-1557.

[41] Oikawa, T., Freeman, M., Lo, W., Vaughan, D.E., and Fogo, A. 1997. Modulation of plasminogen activator inhibitor-1 in vivo: a new mechanism for the anti-fibrotic effect of renin-angiotensin inhibition. *Kidney Int* 51:164-172.

[42] Haraguchi, M., Border, W.A., Huang, Y., and Noble, N.A. 2001. t-PA promotes glomerular plasmin generation and matrix degradation in experimental glomerulonephritis. *Kidney Int* 59:2146-2155.

[43] Keeton, M., Ahn, C., Eguchi, Y., Burlingame, R., and Loskutoff, D.J. 1995. Expression of type 1 plasminogen activator inhibitor in renal tissue in murine lupus nephritis. *Kidney Int* 47:148-157.

[44] Kitching, A.R., Kong, Y.Z., Huang, X.R., Davenport, P., Edgtton, K.L., Carmeliet, P., Holdsworth, S.R., and Tipping, P.G. 2003. Plasminogen activator inhibitor-1 is a significant determinant of renal injury in experimental crescentic glomerulonephritis. *J. Am. Soc. Nephrol.* 14:1487-1495.

[45] Oda, T., Kim, H.S., Wang, D., Lopez-Guisa, J.M., Jernigan, S., and Eddy, A.A. 1999. Effect of genetic PAI-1 deficiency in mice with protein-overload proteinuria [Abstract]. *J. Am. Soc. Nephrol.* 10:578A.

[46] Kim, H., Oda, T., Lopez-Guisa, J., Wing, D., Edwards, D.R., Soloway, P.D., and Eddy, A.A. 2001. TIMP-1 deficiency does not attenuate interstitial fibrosis in obstructive nephropathy. *J. Am. Soc. Nephrol.* 12:736-748.

[47] Edgtton, K.L., Gow, R.M., Kelly, D.J., Carmeliet, P., and Kitching, A.R. 2004. Plasmin is not protective in experimental renal interstitial fibrosis. *Kidney Int* 66:68-76.

[48] Oda, T., Tamura, K., Yoshizawa, N., Sugisaki, T., Matsumoto, K., Hattori, M., Sawai, T., Namikoshi, T., Yamada, M., Kikuchi, Y., et al. 2008. Elevated urinary plasmin activity resistant to alpha2-antiplasmin in acute poststreptococcal glomerulonephritis. *Nephrol. Dial Transplant* 23:2254-2259.

[49] Oda, T., Yamakami, K., Omasu, F., Suzuki, S., Miura, S., Sugisaki, T., and Yoshizawa, N. 2005. Glomerular plasmin-like activity in relation to nephritis-associated plasmin receptor in acute poststreptococcal glomerulonephritis. *J. Am. Soc Nephrol* 16:247-254.

[50] Nicholas, S.B., Aguiniga, E., Ren, Y., Kim, J., Wong, J., Govindarajan, N., Noda, M., Wang, W., Kawano, Y., Collins, A., et al. 2005. Plasminogen activator inhibitor-1 deficiency retards diabetic nephropathy. *Kidney Int* 67:1297-1307.

[51] Collins, S.J., Alexander, S.L., Lopez-Guisa, J.M., Cai, X., Maruvada, R., Chua, S.C., Zhang, G., Okamura, D.M., Matsuo, S., and Eddy, A.A. 2006. Plasminogen activator inhibitor-1 deficiency has renal benefits but some adverse systemic consequences in diabetic mice. *Nephron. Exp. Nephrol.* 104:e23-34.

[52] Hertig, A., Berrou, J., Allory, Y., Breton, L., Commo, F., Costa De Beauregard, M.A., Carmeliet, P., and Rondeau, E. 2003. Type 1 plasminogen activator inhibitor deficiency aggravates the course of experimental glomerulonephritis through overactivation of transforming growth factor beta. *Faseb J.* 17:1904-1906.

[53] Wang, H., Zhang, Y., and Heuckeroth, R.O. 2007. PAI-1 deficiency reduces liver fibrosis after bile duct ligation in mice through activation of tPA. *FEBS Lett* 581:3098-3104.

[54] Eitzman, D.T., McCoy, R.D., Zheng, X., Fay, W.P., Shen, T., Ginsburg, D., and Simon, R.H. 1996. Bleomycin-induced pulmonary fibrosis in transgenic mice that either lack or overexpress the murine plasminogen activator inhibitor-1 gene. *J. Clin. Invest* 97:232-237.

[55] Hattori, N., Degen, J.L., Sisson, T.H., Liu, H., Moore, B.B., Pandrangi, R.G., Simon, R.H., and Drew, A.F. 2000. Bleomycin-induced pulmonary fibrosis in fibrinogen-null mice. *J. Clin. Invest* 106:1341-1350.

[56] Huang, Y., Haraguchi, M., Lawrence, D.A., Border, W.A., Yu, L., and Noble, N.A. 2003. A mutant, noninhibitory plasminogen activator inhibitor type 1 decreases matrix accumulation in experimental glomerulonephritis. *J. Clin. Invest* 112:379-388.

[57] Huang, Y., Border, W.A., Lawrence, D.A., and Noble, N.A. 2006. Noninhibitory PAI-1 enhances plasmin-mediated matrix degradation both in vitro and in experimental nephritis. *Kidney Int* 70:515-522.

[58] Huang, Y., Border, W.A., Yu, L., Zhang, J., Lawrence, D.A., and Noble, N.A. 2008. A PAI-1 mutant, PAI-1R, slows progression of diabetic nephropathy. *J. Am. Soc. Nephrol.* 19:329-338.

[59] Ma, L.J., Nakamura, S., Aldigier, J.C., Rossini, M., Yang, H., Liang, X., Nakamura, I., Marcantoni, C., and Fogo, A.B. 2005. Regression of glomerulosclerosis with high-dose

angiotensin inhibition is linked to decreased plasminogen activator inhibitor-1. *J. Am. Soc. Nephrol.* 16:966-976.

[60] Ma, L.J., Marcantoni, C., Linton, M.F., Fazio, S., and Fogo, A.B. 2001. Peroxisome proliferator-activated receptor-gamma agonist troglitazone protects against nondiabetic glomerulosclerosis in rats. *Kidney Int* 59:1899-1910.

[61] Yu, X., Li, C., Li, X., and Cai, L. 2007. Rosiglitazone prevents advanced glycation end products-induced renal toxicity likely through suppression of plasminogen activator inhibitor-1. *Toxicol Sci.* 96:346-356.

[62] Hoo, R.L., Chow, W.S., Yau, M.H., Xu, A., Tso, A.W., Tse, H.F., Fong, C.H., Tam, S., Chan, L., and Lam, K.S. 2007. Adiponectin mediates the suppressive effect of rosiglitazone on plasminogen activator inhibitor-1 production. *Arterioscler Thromb Vasc. Biol.* 27:2777-2782.

[63] Omasu, F., Oda, T., Yamada, M., Yoshizawa, N., Yamakami, K., Sakurai, Y., and Miura, S. 2007. Effects of pioglitazone and candesartan on renal fibrosis and the intrarenal plasmin cascade in spontaneously hypercholesterolemic rats. *Am. J. Physiol. Renal. Physiol.* 293:F1292-1298.

[64] Benigni, A., Zoja, C., Tomasoni, S., Campana, M., Corna, D., Zanchi, C., Gagliardini, E., Garofano, E., Rottoli, D., Ito, T., et al. 2006. Transcriptional regulation of nephrin gene by peroxisome proliferator-activated receptor-gamma agonist: molecular mechanism of the antiproteinuric effect of pioglitazone. *J. Am. Soc. Nephrol.* 17:1624-1632.

[65] Kanjanabuch, T., Ma, L.J., Chen, J., Pozzi, A., Guan, Y., Mundel, P., and Fogo, A.B. 2007. PPAR-gamma agonist protects podocytes from injury. *Kidney Int.* 71:1232-1239.

In: Nephrology – Dialysis - Transplantation
Editors: Endre Kruger and Kelemen Hahn

ISBN 978-1-60741-736-1
© 2009 Nova Science Publishers, Inc.

Chapter V

Pathogenesis and Resolution Mechanisms of Acute Poststreptococcal Glomerulonephritis

Takashi Oda*[*1] and Nobuyuki Yoshizawa[2]
[1]Department of Nephrology, National Defense Medical College, Saitama
[2]Hemodialysis Unit, Chofu Hospital, Tokyo, Japan

Abstract

Acute poststreptococcal glomerulonephritis (APSGN) develops as an acute nephritic syndrome 1–3 weeks after a streptococcal infection and usually heals without progression. One of the few types of human glomerulonephritis with a clearly defined course of events, it is therefore the appropriate type for which to analyze the process of glomerular injury and resolution. The histological hallmark of this disease in light microscopy is prominent glomerular endocapillary proliferation and in immunofluorescence is granular C3 and/or IgG deposition on the capillary wall. The pathogenic mechanism of APSGN has thus been described by an immune complex theory that involves glomerular deposition of nephritogenic streptococcal antigen and subsequent formation of immune complexes *in situ* and/or the deposition of circulating antigen-antibody complexes. Glomerular immunoglobulin deposition, however, is not often prominent in this disease and the site of glomerular cell infiltration is not the site of immune complex deposition: the major site of inflammation is the inner side of the glomerular tufts, while in early phase of this disease the immune complex is on the outer side of the glomerular tufts. How the nephritogenic antigen induces the glomerular manifestation of APSGN is unknown, and the identity of the causative antigen remains a matter of debate. We recently isolated and characterized a novel nephritogenic antigen of APSGN that we call the nephritis-associated plasmin receptor (NAPlr). It is identical to the plasmin receptor for group A streptococcus and can stabilize and protect plasmin

* Address correspondence to: Takashi Oda, M.D., Department of Nephrology, National Defense Medical College, 3-2 Namiki, Tokorozawa-shi, Saitama 359-8513, Japan Phone: +81-4-2995-1609; Fax: +81-4-2996-5201; E-mail: takashio@ndmc.ac.jp

activity from inhibitors *in vitro*. Glomerular NAPlr deposits are present in essentially all patients with early-phase APSGN. The localization of NAPlr differs from that of C3 or IgG but is almost identical to that of plasmin activity. NAPlr thus has a direct non-immunologic function as a plasmin receptor and might contribute to the pathogenesis of APSGN by maintaining proteolytic activity. Analysis of glomerular hypercellularity revealed that most of the infiltrating cells are macrophages (MΦs) and neutrophils and that a few are CD4+, CD45RO+ T cells. There is a significant positive correlation between the numbers of glomerular infiltrating CD4+ T cells and MΦs. We have also found prominent resident glomerular cell proliferation, particularly in the early phase of APSGN. These histological features suggest that an antigen-specific event related to delayed-type hypersensitivity is involved in the development of APSGN.

We found prominent glomerular cell apoptosis in the early phase of APSGN. The numbers of both proliferating and apoptotic cells decrease exponentially over time, but the decrease is more pronounced for proliferating cells. Thus, apoptosis is predominant in the later phase of the disease and might contribute to the decrease in the number of glomerular cells.

In this chapter our proposed mechanisms of the development and resolution of APSGN are described with special attention to the characteristics of the recently isolated nephritogenic antigen and the contributions of plasmin activity, cell mediated immunity, and apoptosis.

Introduction

Idiopathic glomerulonephritis (GN) is one of the major causes of chronic kidney disease and end-stage renal failure, and its precise pathogenic mechanisms are unknown. Analysis of the onset and the time course of renal disease is crucial for identifying the mechanisms involved but is generally difficult in human GN. The onset and disease course are clear in experimental models, but there are limitations to the application of results in animal models to human conditions considering the biological strain differences.

Acute poststreptococcal glomerulonephritis (APSGN) is a sequel of streptococcus infection and is the prototypic acute nephritic syndrome [1,2]. An atypical asymptomatic form has been recognized [3], but typical APSGN begins in the form of acute nephritic syndrome and usually resolves without progression. Overt APSGN is one of the few types of human GN with a clearly defined course and is thus the appropriate type in which to analyze the processes of glomerular injury and resolution.

Because of the characteristic manifestations of this disease (disease appearance about 1-3 weeks after streptococcal infection, decrement in serum complement titer, and glomerular deposition of C3 and/or IgG in the early phase), it has been widely accepted that the immunological reaction against streptococcus-related antigens is involved in its initiation. The most popular theory of the pathogenic mechanism of APSGN has been the immune complex theory, which involves the glomerular deposition of nephritogenic streptococcal antigen and the subsequent formation of immune complexes *in situ* and/or the deposition of circulating antigen-antibody complexes [1,2]. This theory thus invokes humoral immune mechanisms. Glomerular immunoglobulin deposition, however, is not often prominent in this disease, and the reason for the difference between the site of glomerular cell infiltration and the site of immune complex deposition is unclear: the major site of inflammation is the inner side of the glomerular tufts, whereas in early phase of this disease the immune complex is on the outer side of the glomerular tufts (subepithelial site). Another type of human GN with subepithelial immune complex deposition, membranous nephropathy, is rarely accompanied by endocapillary cell infiltration. Thus, the mechanism of the prominent glomerular endocapillary proliferation occurring in this disease is unknown, and the identity of the causative antigen remains a matter of debate [4–7].

Unlike the development of glomerular injury, the resolution of glomerular damage in humans has been addressed in few reports. This is probably a result of the difficulty of determining the onset point and time course of human GN. This review presents potential mechanisms of the development and resolution of APSGN, with special attention to characteristics of the recently isolated nephritogenic antigen, nephritis-associated plasmin receptor (NAPlr), and to the contributions of plasmin activity, cell mediated immunity, and apoptosis.

Isolation of a Novel Nephritogenic Antigen Related to Plasmin Activity

We isolated a potent nephritogenic antigen from group A streptococcus (GAS) by exploiting its affinity for antibodies in the serum of APSGN patients. A protein fraction was collected from the cytoplasmic proteins of GAS by using affinity chromatography with APSGN patients' IgG-immobilized Sepharose and then purified by ion exchange chromatography. Eventually, a novel 43-kDa protein was isolated [8,9]. The amino acid sequence of the antigen is almost identical to that of the streptococcal plasmin receptor (Plr), also known as glyceraldehyde-3-phosphate dehydrogenase (GAPDH). [8–11], so we call this antigen nephritis-associated plasmin receptor (NAPlr). NAPlr exhibits properties similar to those of Plr, such as specific binding to plasmin(ogen) and GAPDH activity [8]. These findings indicate that even though Plr was isolated from the cell surface fraction and NAPlr was isolated from the cytoplasmic fraction, they are the same molecule.

The following points were examined in order to evaluate the nephritogenicity of the isolated antigen:

1. Whether the antigen accumulates in the affected glomeruli?
2. Whether the antigen induces high levels of antibodies in APSGN patients?
3. Whether the antigen is expressed by nephritis-associated serotypes.?
4. Whether its localization and properties can account for the pathology of APSGN?
5. Whether the antigen can induce nephritis mimicking APSGN in experimental animals?

1. Glomerular Deposition

Figure 1 is the representative photomicrograph of direct immunofluorescence staining for NAPlr with rabbit anti-NAPlr antibody in renal biopsy tissue from an APSGN patient. Prominent NAPlr deposition was found in the glomeruli on mesangial and endocapillary site as ring like pattern. Similar glomerular staining pattern was observed by direct immunofluorescence staining with recently developed mouse monoclonal anti-NAPlr antibody: 1F10 (#ab52322), available from Abcom Inc., Cambridge, MA, USA.

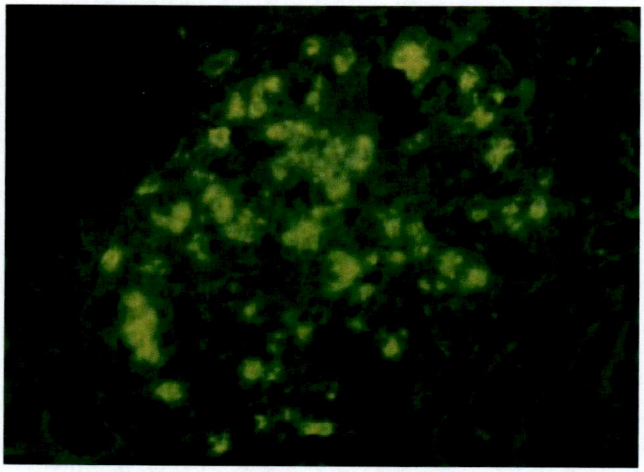

Figure 1. Immunofluorescence staining for NAPlr in tissue sample from a patient with acute poststreptococcal glomerulonephritis. Specific glomerular staining is observed in a ring-like granular pattern.

Table 1. GlomerularNAPlrdeposition in APSGN, non-APSGN and Normal kidney tissues

Biopsy specimens	Onset to biopsy	Glomerular NAPlr (+)	
APSGN	1-14 days	25/25	(100%)
	15-30 days	11/18	(61%)
	31-90 days	0/7	(0%)
	Total	36/50	(72%)
Non-APSGN		4/100	(4%)
Normal kidneys		0/10	(0%)

As shown by the values listed in Table 1, glomerular deposition of NAPlr was observed in 100% (25/25) of APSGN patients within 2 weeks after disease onset or in 84% (36/43) of APSGN patients within 30 days after disease onset by direct immunofluorescence staining with rabbit anti-NAPlr antibody, but the percentage of tissue specimens showing NAPlr deposition decreased over time. On the other hand, no normal kidney was positive for NAPlr and only four of 100 patients with other types of GN were positive for NAPlr [8].

2. Antibody Response

We analyzed the anti-NAPlr antibody titers by Western blotting in serum samples from 50 APSGN patients, 50 streptococcal infection (SI) patients without nephritis, 50 young pediatric patients (<11 years old), 50 older pediatric patients (11–20 years old), 50 young normal adults (25–35 years old), and 50 older normal adults (52–59 years old) [9]. The percentage of those positive for anti-NAPlr antibody was high in APSGN patients and also quite high even in healthy older people (Table 2). APSGN patients, however, showed obviously higher antibody titers than other group, even SI patients without nephritis (Figure 2). Anti-NAPlr antibody titer differed from ASO titer in that the ASO titer was similarly high in both APSGN and SI patients. The anti-NAPlr antibody titer decreased over time but was still higher than normal after 10 years (data not shown). The long-lasting anti-NAPlr antibody might be the reason for the extreme rareness of APSGN recurrence [12].

Table 2. Positive rate of serum anti-NAPlrantibody in patients with APSGN, streptococcal infection, pediatric patients and normal adults

	Age in years range	Anti-NAPlr antibody (+)	
APSGN	5-75 years, mean 29.3	45/50	(90%)
Streptococcal infection	8-64 years, mean 29.0	15/25	(60%)
Pediatric I	0.2-10 years, mean 7.2	13/50	(26%)
Pediatric II	11-20 years, mean 14.1	18/50	(36%)
Normal adults I	25-35 years, mean 30.0	24/50	(48%)
Normal adults II	52-59 years, mean 53.2	36/50	(72%)

3. NAPlr Expression in Nephritogenic Streptococcal Strains

It has been postulated that nephritis is induced by only certain strains of streptococcus [13,14]. To see whether NAPlr would be preferentially expressed in such strains, we analyzed the expression of NAPlr protein and NAPlr mRNA by Western blotting and Northern blotting in various streptococcal strains [15]. Figure 3 shows the Western blotting result. There were essentially no differences in NAPlr expression between streptococcal strains isolated from APSGN patients and strains isolated from non-APSGN patients (pharyngitis patients, scarlet fever patients, toxic shock-like syndrome patients), and similar levels of NAPlr were expressed group A streptococcus (GAS), group C streptococcus (GCS), and group G streptococcus (GGS).

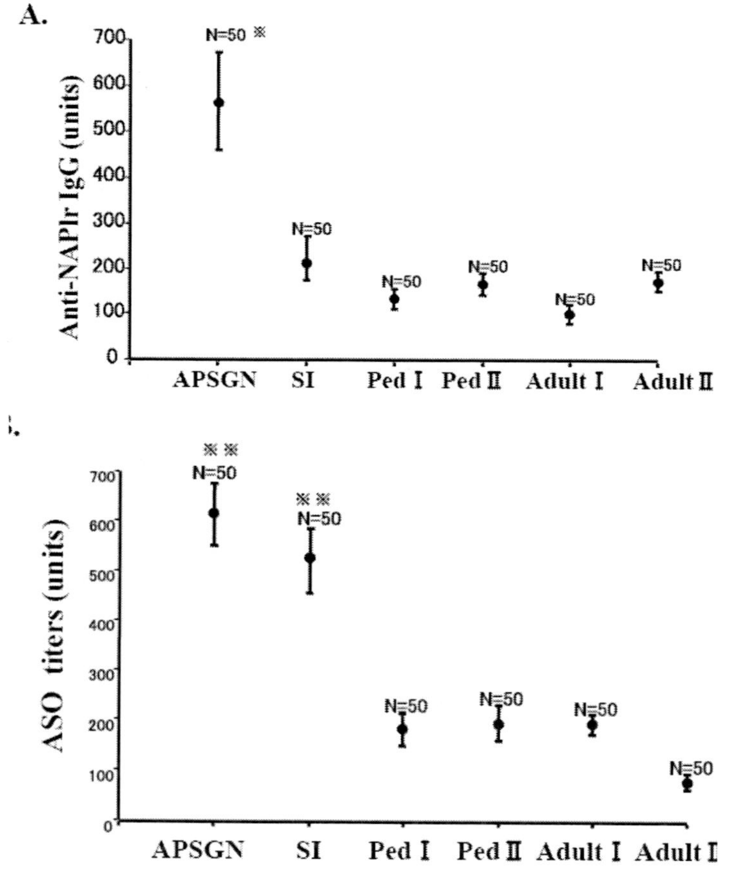

Figure 2. (A) The results of Western blotting assay for anti-NAPlr antibody titers in patients with acute poststreptococcal glomerulonephritis (APSGN), patients with a streptococcal infection (SI) without renal involvement, pediatric patients without renal disease, and normal healthy adults (see Table 1 for ages of subjects in each group). Values are means ± SEM. * $P < 0.05$ for APSGN versus SI, pediatrics, and normal adults by t test. (B) ASO titers for the same groups of patients. The titers in the APSGN and SI groups are significantly higher than those in the normal adults and the pediatric patients without renal disease. Values are means ± SEM. ** $P < 0.001$ for APSGN or SI versus those in other groups by t test.

The mRNA expression assessed by Northern blotting (data not shown) was consistent with the protein expression assessed by Western blotting. Furthermore, the NAPlr gene sequence was highly conserved among these different strains. We thus found no evidence of a specific nephritogenic streptococcal strain, and we suspect that any streptococcal strain can induce nephritis under certain host and bacterial conditions. The candidate nephritogenic antigen streptococcal pyrogenic exotoxin B (SPEB) has also been reported to be found in virtually all *S. pyogenes* isolates [16].

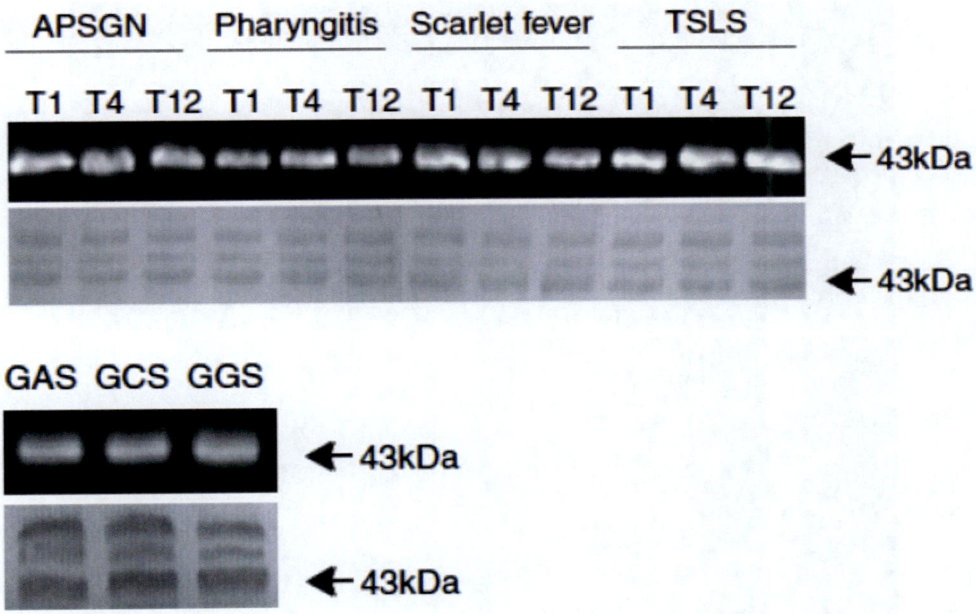

Figure 3. Upper lanes: Western blot analysis of the NAPlr of group A streptococcus from patients with APSGN, pharyngitis, scarlet fever, and toxic shock-like syndrome (TSLS). The apparent 43-kDa protein band which corresponds to NAPlr shows identical amounts of proteins, and these lanes include equal amounts of the proteins. Lower lanes: Western blot analysis of the NAPlr of groups A, C, and G *Streptococci* (GAS, GCS, and GGS). The apparent 43 kDa protein corresponding to NAPlr shows identical amounts of proteins, and these lanes include equal amounts of the proteins.

4. Localization and Properties of Naplr, and Pathogenic Mechanism of APSGN

The important finding with respect to localization of NAPlr was that, as shown for example in Figures 4A–4C, the pattern of NAPlr staining always differed from that of C3 or IgG staining [9]. In early-phase APSGN, C3 and/or IgG deposits are usually found at a subepithelial site (on the outer side of the glomerular tufts), while NAPlr deposits are always found on the inner side of the glomerular tufts. Using double immunofluorescence staining for more precise analysis, we found NAPlr to be localized mainly on the endocapillary neutrophils and mesangial area (Oda *et al.*, manuscript in preparation).

NAPlr is a 43kD protein with a pI of 4.7, and its most characteristic feature *in vitro* is that it binds to plasmin and maintains the proteolytic activity of plasmin by protecting the enzyme from physiological inhibitors such as α_2-antiplasmin (α_2-AP). We found significant glomerular NAPlr deposition in the early phase of APSGN, which led us to speculate that deposited NAPlr would trap plasmin and cause glomerular damage by keeping it in an active condition *in vivo.* To evaluate the feasibility of this hypothesis, we tried to establish the assay for plasmin activity *in situ*.

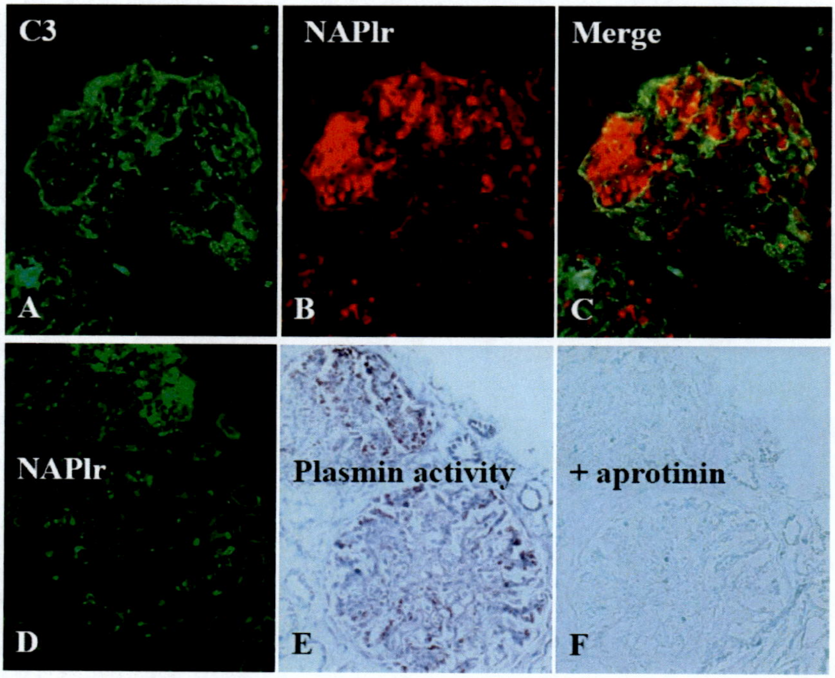

Figure 4. Representative photomicrographs of double immunofluorescence staining for C3 (Alexa Fluor 594; red) and NAPlr (FITC; green) (A–C). The distributions of C3 (A) and NAPlr (B) were obviously different in the merged image (C). (D–F). NAPlr IF staining and *in situ* zymography for plasmin activity in serial sections of renal biopsy tissue from an APSGN patient. The distribution of plasmin activity was similar to that of NAPlr deposition (D, E). Addition of aprotinin inhibited the zymographic activity (F).

Plasminogen is converted to plasmin by two types of plasminogen activators—urokinase type and tissue type—and both types are inhibited by the physiological inhibitor plasminogen activator inhibitor-1 (PAI-1). Plasmin is involved in fibrinolysis, extracellular-matrix turnover, cell migration, wound healing, angiogenesis, and neoplasia [17–20] but because it is easily inhibited and tightly regulated by physiological inhibitors is not normally found in an active form *in vivo.* Using an *in situ* zymography technique with a plasmin-sensitive synthetic substrate (*p*-toluenesulfonyl-L-lysine α-naphthyl ester), we found prominent intraglomerular plasmin activity only in NAPlr-positive APSGN patients (Figure 4E) [21]. This activity was completely inhibited by aprotinin (Figure 4F) but not by α_2-AP. In contrast to the different distributions of NAPlr and C3 or IgG (Figures 4A–4C), the glomerular distributions of plasmin activity and NAPlr are essentially identical (Figures 4D and 4E), suggesting that deposited NAPlr does indeed cause glomerular damage in APSGN by trapping plasmin and maintaining its activity [21]. Plasmin might damage renal tissue directly by degrading extracellular matrix proteins such as fibronectin or laminin but might also exert an indirect effect on extracellular matrix proteins in general by activating pro-matrix metalloproteases [17].

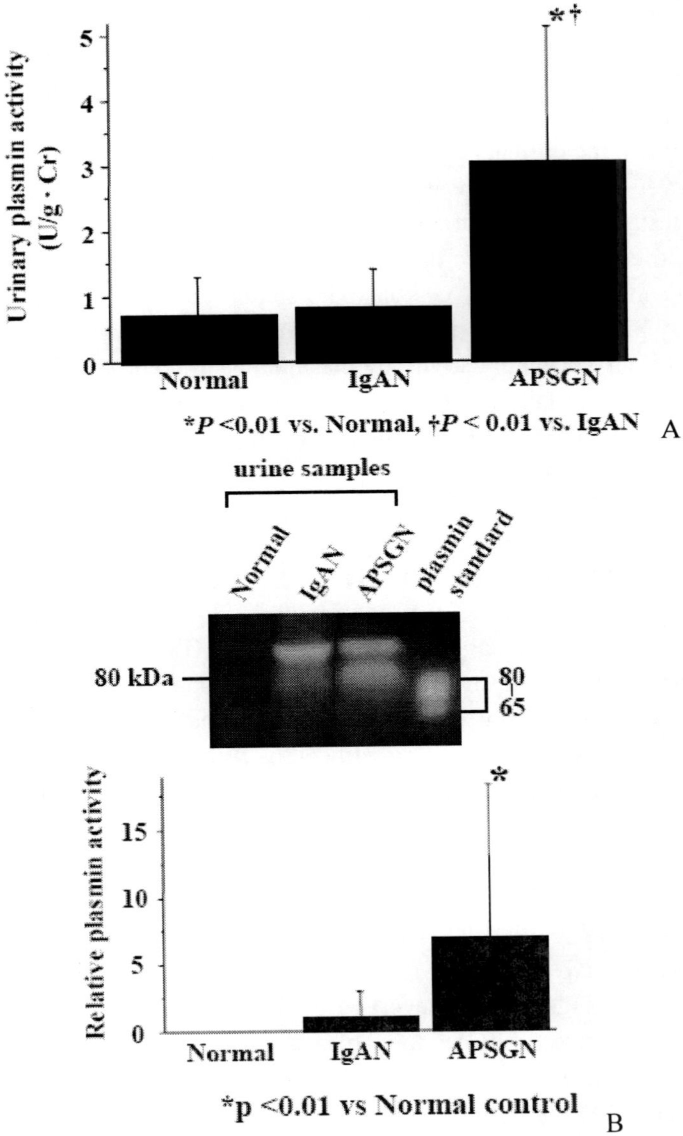

Figure 5. (A). Urinary plasmin activity assessed by chromogenic assay and corrected for urinary creatinine concentration. Results are expressed as corrected mean activity ± SE. *$P < 0.01$ vs. normal control; †$P < 0.01$ vs. IgAN. (B). Representative casein gel zymography results for a plasmin standard and urine supernatants from normal controls, patients with IgAN, and patients with APSGN. Graph shows mean ± SE of the density of 80-kDa bands in casein gel zymography expressed in arbitrary units. *$P < 0.05$ vs. normal controls.

Plasmin can also mediate inflammation by activating monocytes and neutrophils and causing their endothelial accumulation [22,23]. This might account for the different sites of glomerular inflammation and immune-complex deposition in APSGN. NAPlr, putatively maintaining plasmin activity, and the major site of inflammation in APSGN are both endocapillary. Glomerular endocapillary cell infiltration may initially be induced by NAPlr-maintained plasmin activity rather than by subepithelial immune deposits. NAPlr thus acts not only as a component of the immune complex but also as a plasmin receptor and might contribute to the pathogenesis of APSGN by maintaining proteolytic activity. This is consistent with previous clinical findings that proteinuria and microscopic hematuria are occasionally found in the dormant phase of APSGN, when antibody against the nephritogenic antigen has not yet developed. The incidence of APSGN in streptococcal infection patients with these manifestations (proteinuria and hematuria in the dormant phase) is higher than that in streptococcal infection patients without these symptoms [24].

Because the NAPlr-plasmin complex is stable and protected from physiological inhibitors, urinary plasmin activity should be elevated in patients with APSGN. To see if it is, we investigated urinary plasmin activity by plasmin specific chromogenic assay (Figure 5A) and by casein gel zymography (Figure 5B) and found both assays to show that the plasmin activity in the urine of APSGN patients was higher than that in the urine of healthy subjects and IgA nephropathy patients [25].

5. Experimental Animal Models of APSGN

Establishing the experimental animal model of APSGN with the administration of the candidate antigen would be the strongest evidence to support its nephritogenicity. As far as we know, however, there has been no report describing a consistent animal model that reflects human APSGN conditions properly [26–29]. This may probably due to the differential sensitivity of this disease depending on the species or strain differences of the host, as GAS are specific human pathogens.

Despite the above evidence that NAPlr is a potent nephritogenic antigen that could cause APSGN, Batsford *et al.* [30] think that the nephritogenic antigen responsible for APSGN is SPEB, a cationic cysteine protease secreted as a 42-kDa zymogen that is subsequently cleaved to a 28-kDa active proteinase. It is a toxin in severe invasive streptococcal infections [31] but has also been suggested by several groups [4,7,30,32] to be a potent nephritogenic antigen of APSGN. Because of its cationic character, it is suspected to pass easily through the glomerular basement membrane and be deposited at a subepithelial site, where it would then induce immune complex formation. Indeed, Cu *et al.* [7] found glomerular localization of SPEB in 67% of APSGN patients by indirect IF staining with polyclonal anti-SPEB antibody, although they described the localization of SPEB to be endocapillary and in the mesangium of glomeruli. Batsford *et al.* recently compared NAPlr and SPEB in the sera and renal biopsy tissues from a series of APSGN patients with SPEB and streptococcal GAPDH (NAPlr) and associated antibodies that they isolated and/or generated [30]. In contrast to our previous findings [8,9], they found a rare serum antibody response and rare glomerular positivity for streptococcal GAPDH compared to those for SPEB. They therefore argued that SPEB is the principal nephritogenic antigen. However, they used an indirect immunofluorescence staining method with the anti-streptococcal GAPDH antibody that they generated, whereas we performed direct immunofluorescence staining with the anti-NAPlr antibody that we generated. Immunostaining results can vary with the use of different antibodies, so the comparison may be inappropriate [33]. Nonetheless, we compared glomerular localization profiles of SPEB and NAPlr by using an SPEB antibody provided by Dr. Batsford (Department of Immunology, Institute of Medical Microbiology, Freiburg, Germany) and our NAPlr antibody. Double staining showed an extremely similar distribution of both antigens in the glomeruli of APSGN tissues, although NAPlr staining appeared to predominate (most of the SPEB staining being localized within NAPlr-positive areas) [34] (Oda *et al.*, manuscript in preparation). These results were surprising because many researchers have, like us, assumed that there is only one nephritogenic antigen responsible for APSGN. The similar locations of two distinct major antigens in the same glomerulus indicate that this assumption may be incorrect. We should consider the possibility that two or more antigens interact in the development of this disease. In this respect, it is interesting that NAPlr and SPEB are both plasmin-binding antigens and might cause glomerular damage by inducing proteolytic plasmin activity [21,32]. As suggested by Rodriguez-Iturbe [34,35], plasmin activity may be a common final pathway in APSGN.

Cell-Mediated Immunity in APSGN

A prominent increase in the number of endocapillary cells is a histological hallmark of APSGN. Immunohistochemical analysis with various monoclonal antibodies has shown that most of the infiltrating cells are MΦs (CD68+ cells) and neutrophils (chroloesterase+ cells) (Figure 6A) intermingled with a small number of CD4+, CD45RO+ T cells [36,37]. As the duration of the disease increases, the numbers of these cells tends to decrease and the MΦ/neutrophil ratio increases. Furthermore, a significant positive correlation was found between the numbers of glomerular infiltrating CD4+ T cells and MΦs (Figure 6C) [36].

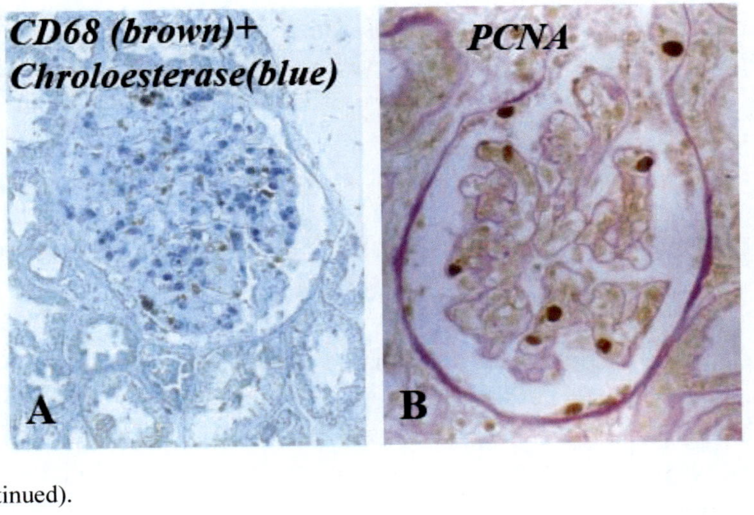

Figure 6. (Continued).

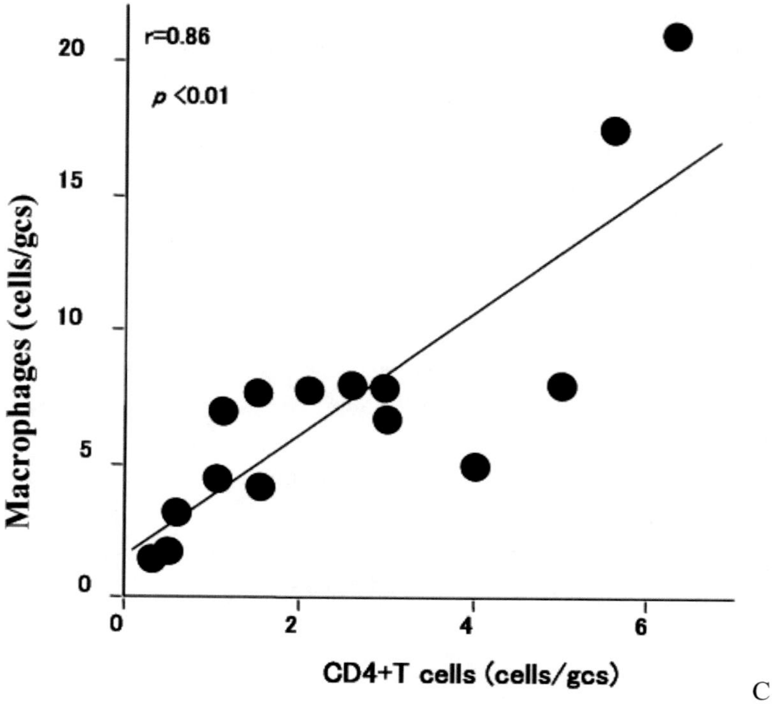

Figure 6. Double staining for chroloesterase (neutrophils, blue) and CD68 (MΦs, brown) (A), and single staining for PCNA with PAS background staining (B) in tissue samples from an APSGN patient. Prominent glomerular infiltration of neutrophils and MΦs (A) and prominent glomerular cell proliferation (B) are evident. There was the significant positive correlation between the numbers of glomerular infiltrating CD4+ cells and macrophages (evaluated as number of cells/ glomerular cross section: gcs) (C).

We also found accelerated resident glomerular cell proliferation, as assessed by proliferating cell nuclear antigen (PCNA) positive cells, particularly in the early phase of this disease (Figure 6B). The majority of proliferating cells in the early phase are endothelial cells; however, as the disease progresses, the number of mesangial cells increases until they constitute nearly half of the proliferating cells within the glomeruli [37]. These histological features suggest that an antigen-specific event related to delayed-type hypersensitivity mediated by helper/inducer T cells is involved in the development of the endocapillary proliferative lesions of APSGN.

Contribution of Apoptosis to the Resolution of APSGN

The development of glomerular injury has been studied extensively, whereas scarcely any data regarding the process of the resolution of glomerular damage are available. APSGN is one of the few types of human GN that usually resolves without progression. We therefore analyzed renal biopsy tissues from APSGN patients with respect to resolution, with attention to the degree of glomerular cell apoptosis and the cell types involved. By terminal deoxynucleotidyl transferase-mediated dUTP nick end-labeling (TUNEL) and immunostaining for single-stranded DNA and caspase-3, we found prominent glomerular cell apoptosis (Figure 7A, B), particularly among glomerular resident cells but also among infiltrating cells (neutrophils and MΦs) [38]. Glomerular cell apoptosis was most prominent in the earliest phase of APSGN, when cell proliferation is also most prominent. The numbers of both proliferating cells and apoptotic cells decrease exponentially over time, but the decrease is more pronounced for proliferating cells (Figure 7C). Glomerular cell apoptosis is thus predominant later in the disease.

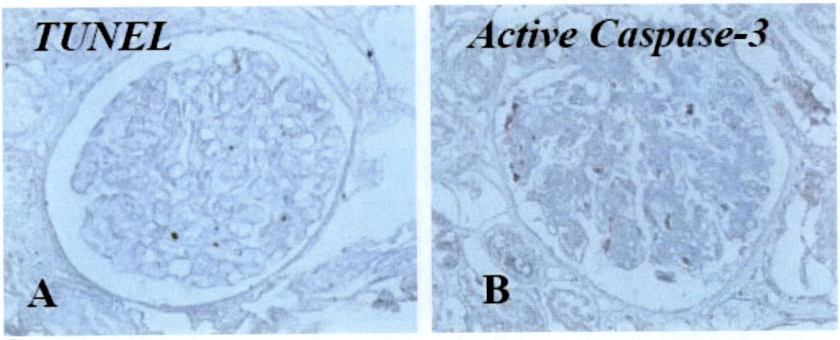

C.

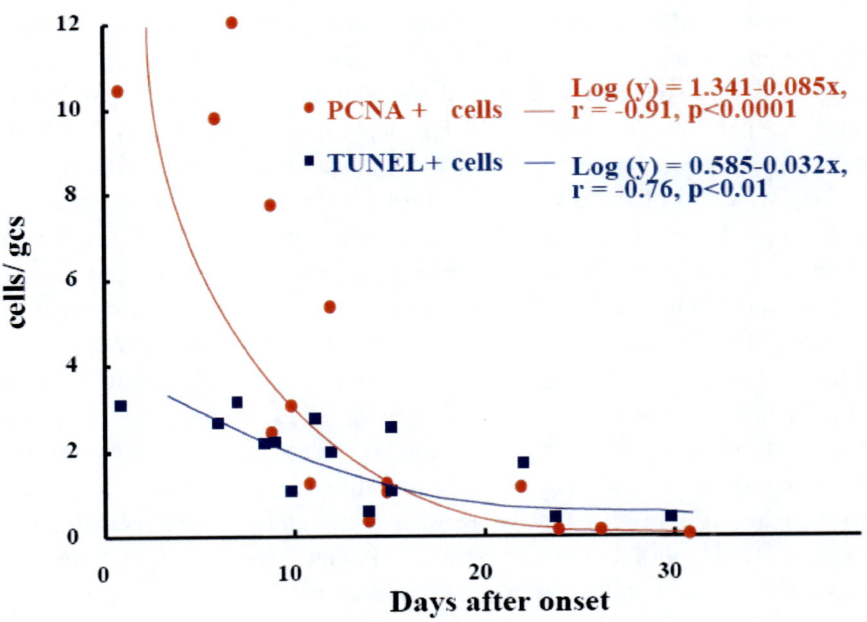

Figure 7. Representative photomicrographs showing increased glomerular cell apoptosis in an APSGN patient by TUNEL (A) and by caspase-3 immunostaining (B). (C): Plot of the numbers of intraglomerular apoptotic (TUNEL+) cells and proliferating (PCNA+) cells (evaluated as number of cells/glomerular cross section: gcs) in APSGN patients against disease duration. The numbers of proliferating cells and apoptotic cells decreased over time and the decrease was slower for the apoptotic cells.

The prominence of cell proliferation and apoptosis evident from the earliest phase of APSGN suggests that the nephritogenic antigen itself may induce proliferation and apoptosis. Most of the apoptotic glomerular cells are indeed within areas of NAPlr deposition [38]. In addition, SPEB has been shown to induce proliferation and apoptosis of human mononuclear leukocytes *in vitro* [39]. As mentioned in the preceding paragraph, the MΦ/neutrophil ratio increases with the duration of the disease, and most of the glomerular MΦs in this disease strongly express the class A macrophage scavenger receptor [38]. These features of infiltrating cells are consistent with the process of resolution of glomerular hypercellularity: scavenger-receptor-mediated phagocytosis by MΦs is a major pathway for the clearance of apoptotic cells [40].

Conclusion

In contrast to the clear clinical features and renal pathology of APSGN, the mechanisms of its development and resolution have not been fully elucidated. In light of our recent finding on nephritogenic antigen responsible for APSGN, we propose the following mechanisms for the development and resolution of APSGN. Infection of the throat or skin with streptococcus induces the release of a nephritogenic antigen, such as NAPlr, into the circulation. Circulating NAPlr accumulates in the renal glomeruli on the mesangial matrix and glomerular basement membrane, probably by adhesion [8]. This NAPlr then traps and maintains the activity of plasmin, which might induce glomerular damage by degrading the glomerular basement membrane by itself or by activating pro-matrix metalloproteases. Plasmin activity may also mediate neutrophil and MΦ infiltration [22,23]. We thus think that an antibody-independent direct effect of the nephritogenic antigen is important for the initiation of the disease. The initial glomerular damage might induce urinary abnormalities during the latent period of the disease. The host immune reaction (both humoral and cell-mediated) against the nephritogenic antigen also develops during this latent period. Cell-mediated immunity, in particular the delayed-type hypersensitivity reactions, contributes to further MΦ accumulation and resident cell proliferation and results in prominent glomerular hypercellularity. The circulating antibody forms immune complexes, either *in situ* or in the circulation that can readily pass through the altered glomerular basement membrane and accumulate in the subepithelial space. These final steps of immune cell accumulation, resident-cell proliferation, and immune complex deposition are accompanied by the activation of complement and lead to the overt disease state. Prominent glomerular cell apoptosis, that are responsible for the resolution of glomerular hypercellularity of this disease, are involved from the earliest phase of APSGN. The lack of a continued supply of NAPlr causes the numbers of proliferating cells and apoptotic cells to decrease over time, and the decrease is more pronounced for the proliferating cells. Apoptosis is thus predominant later in the disease and contributes to the decrease in the number of glomerular cells. Intraglomerular scavenger-receptor-positive MΦs might also contribute by phagocytizing apoptotic cells. The mechanisms localizing NAPlr specifically to the glomeruli and possible contributions and interactions of other nephritic antigens in APSGN must be elucidated in future studies.

Acknowledgments

We are grateful to Dr. Kazuo Yamakami, Department of Preventive Medicine and Public Health, National Defense Medical College, for valuable advice and discussion and to Ms. Tatsuyo Harasawa, Central Research Laboratory, National Defense Medical College, for excellent technical assistance.

References

[1] Couser WG, Johnson RJ: Postinfectious glomerulonephritis. *Immunologic renal diseases.* Edited by Neilson EG, Couser WG. Philadelphia, Lippincott-Raven, 1997, pp 915-943

[2] Silva FG: Acute postinfectious glomerulonephritis and glomerulonephritis complicating persistent bacterial infection. *Heptinstall's Pathology of the Kidney.* Edited by Jennette JC, Olson JL, Schwartz MM, Silva FG. Philadelphia, Lippincott-Raven, 1998, pp 389-453.

[3] Yoshizawa N, Suzuki Y, Oshima S, Takeuchi A, Kondo S, Ishida A, Nakabayashi I, Nishiyama J, Tazawa K, Sagel I: Asymptomatic acute poststreptococcal glomerulonephritis following upper respiratory tract infections caused by Group A streptococci. *Clin. Nephrol.* 1996, 46:296-301.

[4] Vogt A, Batsford S, Rodriguez-Iturbe B, Garcia R: Cationic antigens in poststreptococcal glomerulonephritis. *Clin. Nephrol.* 1983, 20:271-279.

[5] Lange K, Seligson G, Cronin W: Evidence for the in situ origin of poststreptococcal glomerulonephritis: glomerular localization of endostreptosin and the clinical significance of the subsequent antibody response. *Clin. Nephrol.* 1983, 19:3-10.

[6] Johnston KH, Zabriskie JB: Purification and partial characterization of the nephritis strain-associated protein from Streptococcus pyogenes, group A. *J. Exp. Med.* 1986, 163:697-712.

[7] Cu GA, Mezzano S, Bannan JD, Zabriskie JB: Immunohistochemical and serological evidence for the role of streptococcal proteinase in acute post-streptococcal glomerulonephritis. *Kidney Int* 1998, 54:819-826.

[8] Yamakami K, Yoshizawa N, Wakabayashi K, Takeuchi A, Tadakuma T, Boyle MD: The potential role for nephritis-associated plasmin receptor in acute poststreptococcal glomerulonephritis. *Methods* 2000, 21:185-197.

[9] Yoshizawa N, Yamakami K, Fujino M, Oda T, Tamura K, Matsumoto K, Sugisaki T, Boyle MD: Nephritis-associated plasmin receptor and acute poststreptococcal glomerulonephritis: characterization of the antigen and associated immune response. *J. Am. Soc. Nephrol.* 2004, 15:1785-1793.

[10] Lottenberg R, Broder CC, Boyle MD, Kain SJ, Schroeder BL, Curtiss R, 3rd: Cloning, sequence analysis, and expression in Escherichia coli of a streptococcal plasmin receptor. *J. Bacteriol.* 1992, 174:5204-5210.

[11] Winram SB, Lottenberg R: The plasmin-binding protein Plr of group A streptococci is identified as glyceraldehyde-3-phosphate dehydrogenase. *Microbiology* 1996, 142 (Pt 8):2311-2320.

[12] Watanabe T, Yoshizawa N: Recurrence of acute poststreptococcal glomerulonephritis. *Pediatr. Nephrol.* 2001, 16:598-600.

[13] Rammelkamp CH, Jr., Weaver RS: Acute glomerulonephritis, the significance of the variations in the incidence of the disease. *J. Clin. Invest* 1953, 32:345-358.

[14] Bisno AL, Pearce IA, Wall HP, Moody MD, Stollerman GH: Contrasting epidemiology of acute rheumatic fever and acute glomerulonephritis. *N. Engl. J. Med.* 1970, 283:561-565.

[15] Fujino M, Yamakami K, Oda T, Omasu F, Murai T, Yoshizawa N: Sequence and expression of NAPlr is conserved among group A streptococci isolated from patients with acute poststreptococcal glomerulonephritis (APSGN) and non-APSGN. *J. Nephrol.* 2007, 20:364-369.

[16] Rodriguez-Iturbe B, Batsford S: Pathogenesis of poststreptococcal glomerulonephritis a century after Clemens von Pirquet. *Kidney Int* 2007, 71:1094-1104.

[17] Vassalli JD, Sappino AP, Belin D: The plasminogen activator/plasmin system. *J. Clin. Invest* 1991, 88:1067-1072.

[18] Mignatti P, Rifkin DB: Biology and biochemistry of proteinases in tumor invasion. *Physiol. Rev.* 1993, 73:161-195.

[19] Eitzman DT, Ginsburg D: Of mice and men. The function of plasminogen activator inhibitors (PAIs) in vivo. *Adv. Exp. Med. Biol.* 1997, 425:131-141.

[20] Oda T, Jung YO, Kim HS, Cai X, Lopez-Guisa JM, Ikeda Y, Eddy AA: PAI-1 deficiency attenuates the fibrogenic response to ureteral obstruction. Kidney Int 2001, 60:587-596.

[21] Oda T, Yamakami K, Omasu F, Suzuki S, Miura S, Sugisaki T, Yoshizawa N: Glomerular plasmin-like activity in relation to nephritis-associated plasmin receptor in acute poststreptococcal glomerulonephritis. *J. Am. Soc. Nephrol.* 2005, 16:247-254.

[22] Montrucchio G, Lupia E, De Martino A, Silvestro L, Savu SR, Cacace G, De Filippi PG, Emanuelli G, Camussi G: Plasmin promotes an endothelium-dependent adhesion of neutrophils. Involvement of platelet activating factor and P-selectin. *Circulation* 1996, 93:2152-2160.

[23] Burysek L, Syrovets T, Simmet T: The serine protease plasmin triggers expression of MCP-1 and CD40 in human primary monocytes via activation of p38 MAPK and janus kinase (JAK)/STAT signaling pathways. *J. Biol. Chem.* 2002, 277:33509-33517.

[24] Nissenson AR, Baraff LJ, Fine RN, Knutson DW: Poststreptococcal acute glomerulonephritis: fact and controversy. Ann. Intern Med 1979, 91:76-86.

[25] Oda T, Tamura K, Yoshizawa N, Sugisaki T, Matsumoto K, Hattori M, Sawai T, Namikoshi T, Yamada M, Kikuchi Y, Suzuki S, Miura S: Elevated urinary plasmin activity resistant to alpha2-antiplasmin in acute poststreptococcal glomerulonephritis. *Nephrol. Dial Transplant* 2008, 23:2254-2259.

[26] Lindberg LH, Vosti KL, Raffel S: Experimental streptococcal glomerulonephritis in rats. *J. Immunol.* 1967, 98:1231-1240.

[27] Becker CG, Murphy GE: The experimental induction of glomerulonephritis like that in man by infection with group A streptococci. *J. Exp. Med.* 1968, 127:1-24.

[28] Markowitz AS, Horn D, Aseron C, Novak R, Battiforia HA: Streptococcal related glomerulonephritis. 3. Glomerulonephritis in rhesus monkeys immunologically induced both actively and passively with a soluble fraction from nephritogenic streptococcal protoplasmic membranes. *J. Immunol.* 1971, 107:504-511.

[29] Yoshizawa N, Oshima S, Takeuchi A, Kondo S, Oda T, Shimizu J, Nishiyama J, Ishida A, Nakabayashi I, Tazawa K, Sakurai Y: Experimental acute glomerulonephritis induced in the rabbit with a specific streptococcal antigen. *Clin. Exp. Immunol.* 1997, 107:61-67.

[30] Batsford SR, Mezzano S, Mihatsch M, Schiltz E, Rodriguez-Iturbe B: Is the nephritogenic antigen in post-streptococcal glomerulonephritis pyrogenic exotoxin B (SPE B) or GAPDH? *Kidney Int* 2005, 68:1120-1129.

[31] Nagamune H, Ohkura K, Ohkuni H: Molecular basis of group A streptococcal pyrogenic exotoxin B. *J. Infect Chemother*. 2005, 11:1-8.

[32] Poon-King R, Bannan J, Viteri A, Cu G, Zabriskie JB: Identification of an extracellular plasmin binding protein from nephritogenic streptococci. *J. Exp. Med.* 1993, 178:759-763.

[33] Yoshizawa N, Yamakami K, Oda T: Nephritogenic antigen for acute poststreptococcal glomerulonephritis. *Kidney Int* 2006, 69:942-943; author reply 942.

[34] Rodriguez-Iturbe B, Musser JM: The current state of poststreptococcal glomerulonephritis. *J. Am. Soc. Nephrol.* 2008, 19:1855-1864.

[35] Rodriguez-Iturbe B: Nephritis-associated streptococcal antigens: where are we now? *J. Am. Soc Nephrol.* 2004, 15:1961-1962.

[36] Yoshizawa N, Oda T, Oshikawa Y, Akashi Y, Suzuki Y, Shimizu J, Shimizu E, Niwa H, Treser G: Cell-mediated immune response in acute poststreptococcal glomerulonephritis. *Nippon Jinzo Gakkai Shi* 1994, 36:322-330.

[37] Oda T, Yoshizawa N, Takeuchi A, Nakabayashi I, Nishiyama J, Ishida A, Tazawa K, Murayama M, Hotta O, Taguma Y: Glomerular proliferating cell kinetics in acute post-streptococcal glomerulonephritis (APSGN). *J. Pathol.* 1997, 183:359-368.

[38] Oda T, Yoshizawa N, Yamakami K, Ishida A, Hotta O, Suzuki S, Miura S: Significance of glomerular cell apoptosis in the resolution of acute post-streptococcal glomerulonephritis. *Nephrol. Dial Transplant* 2007, 22:740-748.

[39] Viera NT, Romero MJ, Montero MK, Rincon J, Mosquera JA: Streptococcal erythrogenic toxin B induces apoptosis and proliferation in human leukocytes. *Kidney Int* 2001, 59:950-958.

[40] Savill J, Smith J, Sarraf C, Ren Y, Abbott F, Rees A: Glomerular mesangial cells and inflammatory macrophages ingest neutrophils undergoing apoptosis. *Kidney Int* 1992, 42:924-936.

In: Nephrology – Dialysis - Transplantation
Editors: Endre Kruger and Kelemen Hahn
ISBN 978-1-60741-736-1
© 2009 Nova Science Publishers, Inc.

Chapter VI

Progression of Autossomal Dominant Polycystic Kidney Disease: A Follow-Up Study of a Large Cohort in a Single Center

Edgar A. F. de Almeida, José António Lopes, M. Martins Prata and A. Gomes da Costa
Serviço de Nefrologia e Transplantação Renal,
Centro Hospitalar Lisboa Norte, EPE, Lisboa, Portugal

Abstract

Autosomal Dominant Polycystic Kidney Disease (ADPKD) is the cause of renal failure in 5-10% of the patients in dialysis or transplantation. Several conditions are associated to the rate of progression. In this manuscript we presented data on the rate of progression of a large cohort of patients followed in a single institution by a one and only nephrologist for a mean time of 95 months.

Methods: 420 patients (178 males; 360 with a positive family history) were regularly seen in outpatient setting since 1989, the mean follow-up was 95,0 ± 64,4 months [median 85, range 2-353] and the mean number of visits was 15,4 ± 11,3 [median 12, range 1-55 visits]. In each visit analysis of the renal function, blood pressure and relevant clinical data were registered. The rate of progression to chronic renal failure (CRF) was evaluated using Kaplan-Meier (KM) survival analysis. Additionally we compared the slope of the regression line of the 1/serum creatinine versus time plot (PLOT) as well as the rate of deterioration of creatinine clearance, calculated by Cockroft-Gault formula (CGF), in 226 patients with a minimum follow-up of 60 months and 6 visits.

Results: Mean age of renal death was 56,1 ± 11,9 years in men as compared to 57,8 ± 12,7 in women (p=ns); KM survival curves showed that 50% of the men started dialysis by the age of 65,8 while women started at 69,8 years (95% CI: 62,1-69,4; log rank 2,88; p=0,08). Similarly, no differences were found between patients who inherited the disease from their father and those who inherited from their mothers. Patients with mean office blood pressure (MAP) higher than 106 had worse renal prognosis (log-rank

4,2; $p<0,04$). Patients who had haematuria ($p<0,001$) or who had any urologic symptoms (haematuria, renal colic or cyst infection) had considerably worse prognosis than those whose follow-up was uneventful ($p<0,02$). As ascertained by the slope of PLOT, patients with fast progression (slope $< -0,0043$), more had initiated dialysis ($p<0,001$), had more haematuria ($p<0,001$), higher MAP ($p<0,001$) and a higher rate of deterioration of CGF ($p<0,001$) than those with slow progression (slope $> 0,001$). Similarly, patients with CGF rate greater than 4,27 ml/min/year (fast progressors) are older, more had started dialysis, had more haematuria, higher MAP and steeper slope in the PLOT analysis.

Conclusions: ADPKD patients with urologic symptoms and higher blood pressure had increased risk for progression to CRF.

Introduction

Autosomal dominant polycystic kidney disease (ADPKD) is one of the most common hereditary diseases in adults [1]. The prevalence of ADPKD is estimated as 1: 500 to 1: 2500 in western countries and contributes to a substantial number of patients in renal replacement therapies (RRT). Although children may present cardiovascular symptoms the disease characteristically appears in adults. The emergence of hypertension in the third decade of life as well as urologic manifestations such as renal colic, nephrolithiasis and haematuria is the hallmark of ADPKD in adults. In some families cerebral aneurisms are ominous signs as they impose a serious threat to life. However patients with ADPKD are mostly concerned with the progressive nature of the disease as the need for renal replacement therapy may occur as early as in the fourth decade of life.

In the past 25 years considerable amount of knowledge has been gathered on the genetic origin of the disease. ADPKD is the result of a mutation in two different genes, PKD1 on the short arm of chromosome 16 coding for polycystin 1, and PKD2 on the long arm of chromosome 4 coding for polycystin 2 [2]. The existence of other loci cannot be excluded as absence of linkage to either PKD1 or PKD2 loci was found in some families [3]. It was shown that polycystin 1 and polycystin 2 participate in several cellular functions that regulate cellular proliferation, differentiation and fate, and these functions are important in early stages of tubulogenesis and renal morphogenesis [4].

Progression to end-stage renal disease occurs in a significant number of patients irrespective of the medical or dietary interventions. Several studies addressing the risk factors for faster progression in ADPKD patients demonstrated that families carrying PKD1 mutations had a worse prognosis than those with PKD2 mutations. In fact, there is a significant difference in the age of initiation of renal replacement therapy between these two groups and, therefore, the genotype is the most powerful predictor factor of faster progression [5]. Several other clinical parameters have been evaluated as risk factor for progression such as gender, blood pressure control, hepatic cysts, haematuria, proteinuria and urologic manifestations [6-9]. In the current study, a large cohort of patients with one of the largest follow-up and always treated by a single nephrologist was evaluated for these risk factors.

Population and Methods

Between 1979 and September 2008 more than 500 patients with bilateral renal cysts were observed in an outpatient setting at the Nephrology Department at the Hospital de Santa Maria, Lisbon, Portugal. Patients were referred by other clinicians such as general practitioners, urologists and internists due to the presence of renal cysts in a renal scan, hypertension, urologic symptoms or renal failure. A considerable amount of patients were first diagnosed by us in a screening project of at risk first-degree relatives. Screening was proposed to first-degree relatives older than 18 and after counselling. However several patients were diagnosed earlier due to the occurrence of abdominal symptoms that prompted the use of ultrasound scans or even in ultrasound scans performed during pregnancy.

Patients were followed-up in an outpatient setting at least in a yearly basis but more often if necessary. In each visit all occurrences were registered particularly those related with blood pressure control and urologic symptoms such as macroscopic haematuria, urinary tract infection, renal colic and nephrolithiasis. Renal function tests (serum urea and serum creatinine) as well as blood pressure and body weight were also registered in each visit. Medication for blood pressure control or other comorbidities (statins, for example) were adjusted and patients were counselled about nephroprotective measures such as diet, water ingestion, and avoiding nephrotoxic such as non-steroidal anti-inflammatory.

Diagnostic criteria for ADPKD were those proposed by Bear [10], e.g., bilateral involvement of the kidneys at least with 3 cysts and a positive family history for ADPKD. Applying the above criteria 360 patients (149 male) were diagnosed as ADPKD and constituted Group 1. Patients with renal and hepatic cysts in absence of family history were considered as having putative PKD and constituted Group 2 (n=60; 29 male). Patients with simple renal cysts in absence of hepatic cysts and family history were excluded from further analysis. In-office blood pressure measurements were performed after 5 minutes in sitting position and mean blood pressure (MAP) was calculated as the sum of diastolic blood pressure to 1/3 of the difference between systolic and diastolic blood pressure. For each patient the average of all MAP measured in each visit was quoted and this figure was considered as the office blood pressure (aMBP).

In patients with a minimum follow-up of 60 months and at least 6 determinations of the serum creatinine, the rate of progression of renal failure was estimated by the slope of the regression line of the 1/serum creatinine versus time plot and by estimation of glomerular filtration rate using the Cockroft-Gault formula [11]. For each patient this estimation was done in each visit and the evolution of eGFR was evaluated using an eGFR versus time plot. A regression line was inferred and the equation obtained was used to calculate the rate of deterioration of the renal function in ml/min/year.

Kaplan-Meier Survival Analysis

The age at initiation of dialysis was assumed as the measure of the rate of progression to end-stage renal disease. Therefore, time to initiation of dialysis in months (or time to death) was computed using the Kaplan-Meier method. Lost to follow-up was also censored. Log-rank test was employed to determine statistically differences between the curves. The effect of covariates on time to initiation of dialysis was evaluated using the Cox proportions hazard method. A two-tailed p<0,05 was assumed as significant.

Results

Four hundred and twenty patients (178 men) were included in the analysis, 60 of them (29 men) no family history of ADPKD or chronic renal failure was established. Thirty-five patients were observed only once at the initiation of the renal replacement therapy (RRT), and were included only in the survival analysis comparing the influence of gender and affected progenitor. Of the remaining 385 patients (161 men; 224 women) the mean follow-up time was 95,0 ± 64,4 months [7,9 years] (median 85; range 1-353 months [29,4 years]). The mean number of visits was 15,4 ± 11,3 (median 12 visits; range 1-55).

At the span of the follow-up period 48 patients (15 men; 33 women) were lost to follow-up and were censored at the time of the last visit. Similarly, 4 patients died (1 men; 3 women) before the initiation of RRT; 2 patients died from cardiovascular disease and 2 due to malignant neoplasms. In the duration of the follow-up period 117 patients (57 men; 60 women) started RRT, either hemodialysis or peritoneal dialysis. None received pre-emptive renal transplantation.

The Effect of Gender on Renal Progression

Mean age at the initiation of RRT was 56,1 ± 11,9 years in men, slightly younger than in women 57,8 ± 12,7 years, although not statistically significant (p=0,2). Assuming age at the initiation of RRT or death as endpoint, Kaplan-Meier survival analysis showed that 50% of men started RRT by the age of 65,8 while 50% of the women started at 69,8 years (95% CI: 62,1-69,4; log rank 2,88; p=0,08) [Figure 1]. Similarly, no differences were found when the slopes of the 1/scr of the 93 men and 133 women whose follow-up were longer than 5 years and had 6 or more observations were compared (mean slope -0,0023 ± 0,004 versus -0,0018 ± 0,0031; p=ns). However, men showed faster progression as evaluated by the rate of deterioration of the eGFR (2,76 ± 2,83 versus 1,65 ± 4,18 ml/min/year; p<0,04).

The Effect of Parental Origin of the Gene

Parental origin of the gene was known in 280 subjects. In 115 patients the origin of the gene was his/her father and in 165 the patient inherited the gene from his/her mother. Kaplan-Meier analysis showed no differences when patients who inherited the disease from their father were compared to those who inherited the disease from their mother (Figure 2). The age at which 50% of the patients started RRT was 62 years for those who inherited the disease from their father and 67 years for those who inherited from their mother.

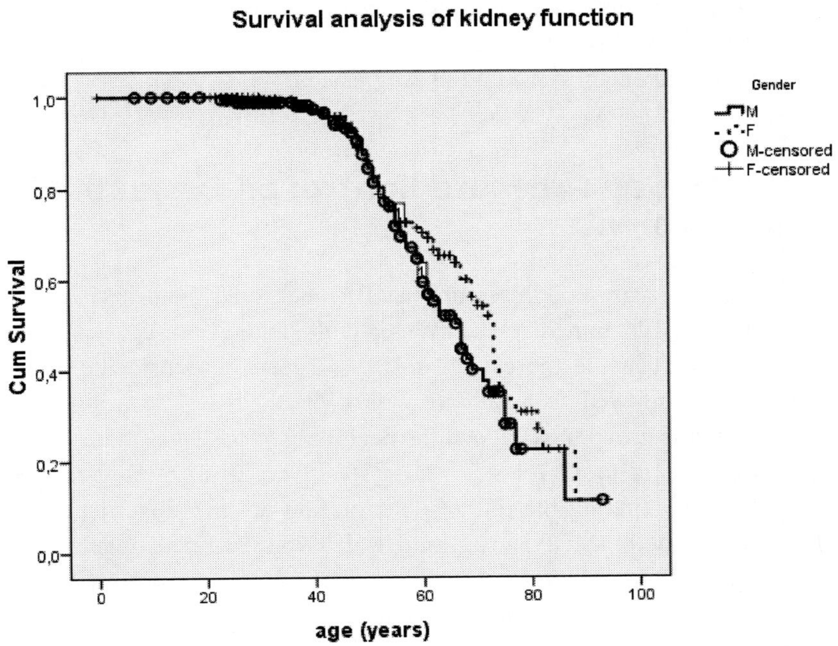

Figure 1. Kaplan-Meier survival analysis comparing the effect of gender (M- male; F – female) in the progression of ADPKD.

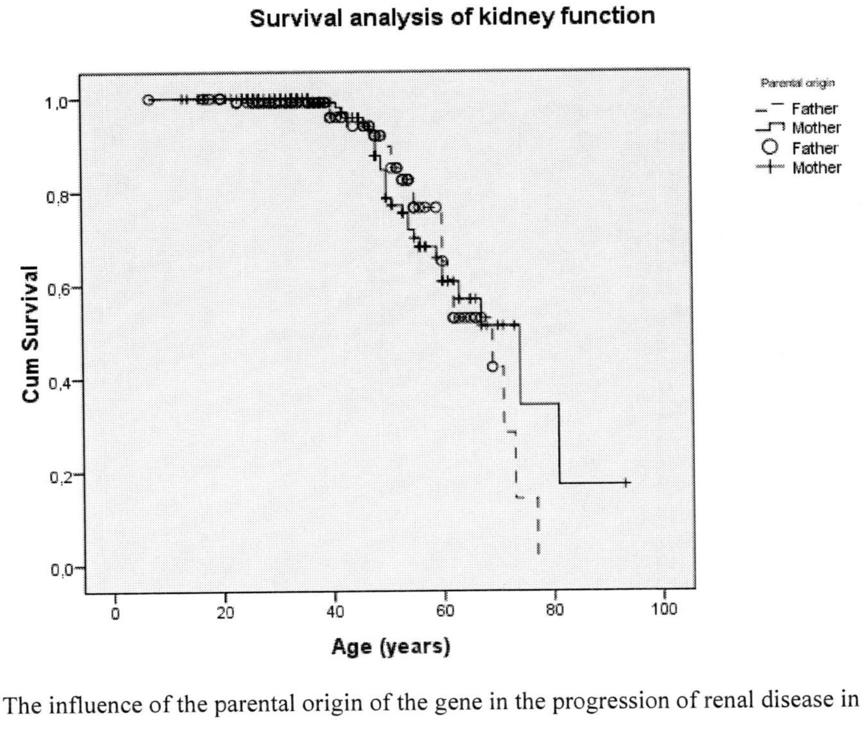

Figure 2. The influence of the parental origin of the gene in the progression of renal disease in ADPKD.

The same results were obtained using the slope of the 1/scr or the rate of deterioration of eGFR. Moreover, father to son and father to daughter as well as mother to son and mother to daughter showed no differences in the rate of progression.

The Effect of Blood Pressure Control as Evaluated by in-Office Measurements

The average of the mean blood pressure (aMBP) measured in each visit was computed. Patients with aMBP < 106 mm of mercury (<140/90 mmHg) were considered as having controlled blood pressure while those with aMBP ≥ 106 were considered as uncontrolled. Kaplan-Meier analysis showed that patients with aMBP ≥ 106 had a significantly worse prognosis. In fact, in this group mean age at the beginning of RRT was 67,2 ± 1,8 years (95% CI 63,6-70,8) as compared to 77,1 ± 2,7 years (95% CI 71,6-82,6) [log-rank 4,2; p<0,04] (Figure 3). Similarly, comparing the rate of deterioration of renal function and the slope of the 1/scr plot, patients with aMBP > 106 mmHg deteriorated renal function faster (2,79 ± 3,64 versus 1,58 ± 3,72 ml/min/year; p<0,03) and had a steeper slope (-0,0027 ± 0,0041 versus -0,0015 ± 0,0034; p< 0,03) than those with controlled blood pressure. Besides, those who started RRT did it at a younger age if aMBP > 106 (52,3 ± 10,1 versus 58,0 ± 12,5 years; p<0,05). After adjusting for covariates, aMBP (adjusted hazard ratio 1,05; 95% CI 1,00-1,10; p<0,03) emerged as an important risk factor for progression to chronic renal failure.

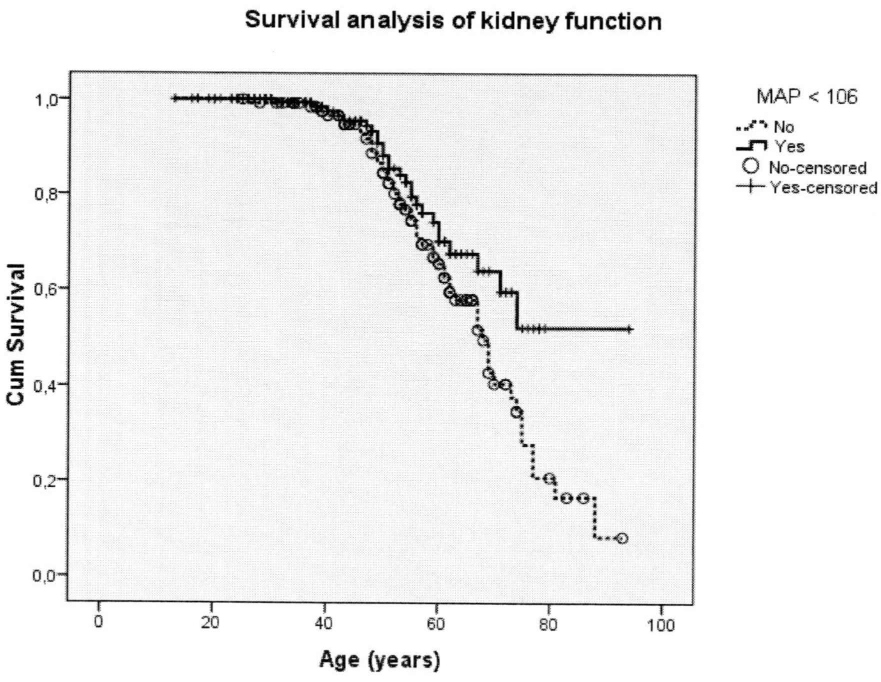

Figure 3. The effect of blood pressure control on kidney function.

The Effect of Gross Haematuria

Gross haematuria, not associated with urinary tract infection or renal colic, was reported in 90 of 326 patients with follow-up. When compared to those who hadn't haematuria they had a worse renal fate. In fact, 50% of the patients with haematuria started RRT by the age of 59 years compared to 69 years in those without haematuria (log-rank 13,01; $p<0,001$) (Figure 4). Patients with haematuria have a faster deterioration of the renal function ($3,60 \pm 3,25$ versus $1,67 \pm 4,91$ ml/min/year; $p<0,002$) and steeper slope of the 1/scr plot ($-0,0037 \pm 0,0033$ versus $-0,0018 \pm 0,0049$; $p< 0,001$).

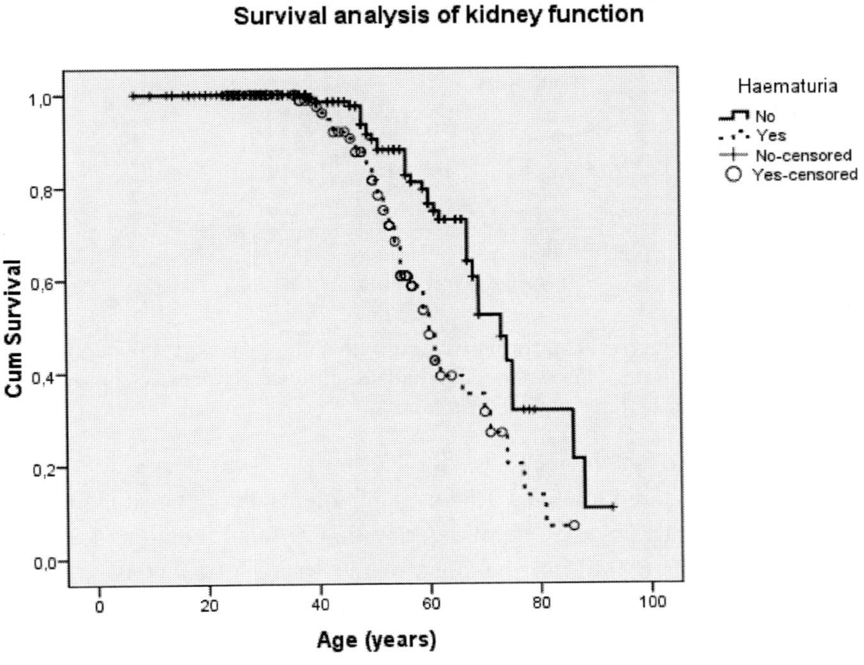

Figure 4. Patients with history of gross haematuria exhibit a worse renal prognosis when compared with those who didn´t report haematuria.

The Effect of Urinary Tract Infection and Cyst Infection

During the follow-up 58 patients (9 men) reported at least one episode of cystitis (23 of them had more than 1 episode). Although they were told to perform urine microbiology before the initiation of antibiotics, data on the results of urine analysis are scarce. Comparing the outcome of patients with episodes of cystitis with those who did not experienced it no differences were found in Kaplan-Meier survival analysis neither on the rate of deterioration of renal function nor on the slope of the 1/scr plot. If separate analysis is performed, men had a worse renal prognosis, although not statistically significant ($p=0,08$), if they suffered urinary tract infection. However, the outcome of the 20 patients who had cyst infection is significantly poor when compared to rest of the population (Figure 5).

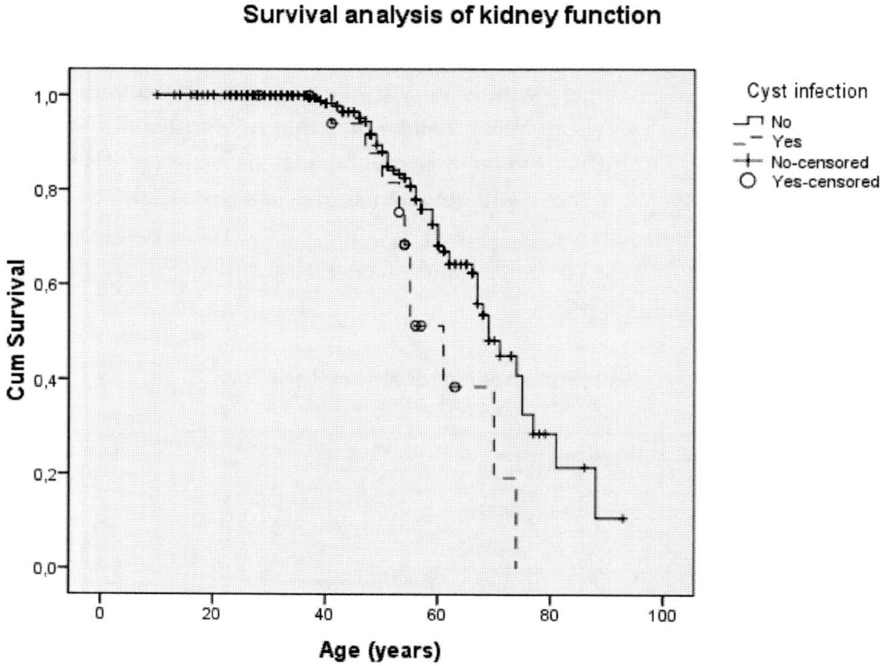

Figure 5. Cumulative renal survival comparing patients with and without cyst infection during the follow-up. Patients with episodes of cysts infection had a significantly worse renal prognosis as evaluated by the age of starting renal replacement therapy.

In Kaplan-Meier analysis the mean age for starting RRT was 60,4 ± 2,9 years in patients with cyst infections compared to 69,8 ± 1,8 years in patients without cyst infection. The same results were obtained analysing the rate of deterioration of renal function (4,27 ± 3,84 versus 2,09 ± 4,59 ml/min/year; p<0,05) or the slope of the 1/scr plot (-0,0041 ± 0,0034 versus -0,0022 ± 0,0046; p<0,05).

The Effect of Renal Colic

Renal colic as a surrogate for neprolithiasis was experienced by 115 patients along the duration of the follow-up. No differences were found when patients with history of renal colic were compared to those without renal colic neither in Kaplan-Meier survival analysis nor in the rate of deterioration of renal function and in the slope of 1/scr plot.

Urologic Manifestation and the Rate of Progression

If those who had experienced any urologic manifestation, such as haematuria, renal colic, urinary tract infection or cyst infection, are compared to those who were free of these symptoms, no differences were found in Kaplan-Meier survival analysis. However, man with urologic symptoms had a significantly worse prognosis than those who were free (Figure 6).

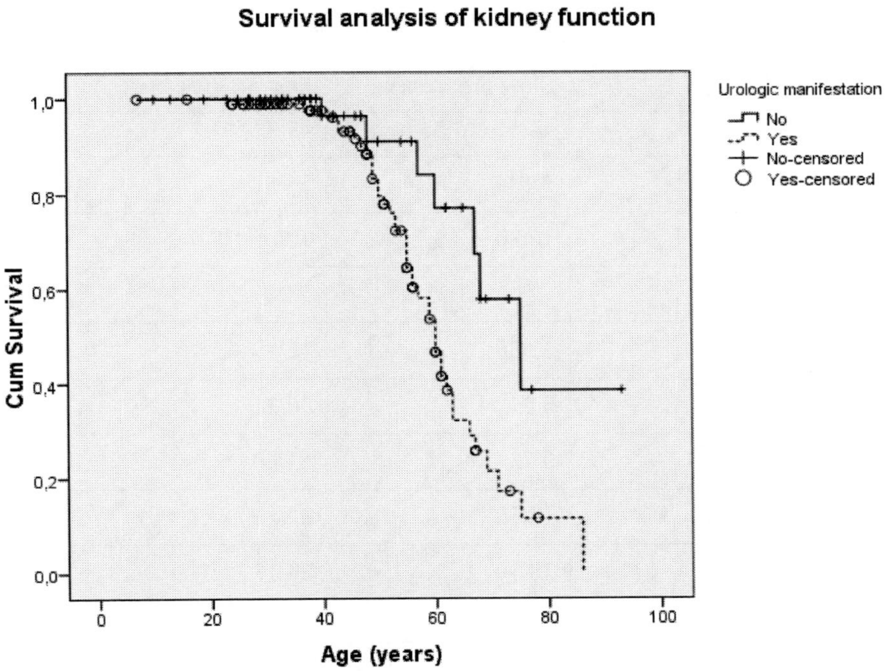

Figure 6. Kaplan-Meier survival analysis of the age at initiation of renal replacement therapy in ADPKD men with or without urologic symptoms.

In fact, the mean survival time of men with urologic symptoms is significantly lower (61,1 ± 1,8 years; 95% CI 56,6 -63,3 versus 75,4 ± 4,7 years; 95% CI 66,2 – 84,7; p<0,01). After adjusting for covariates urologic symptoms (adjusted hazard ratio 6,3; 95% CI 1,61-24,7; p<0,01) emerged as an important risk factor for progression to chronic renal failure.

Fast and Slow Progressors

Slope of the 1/scr plot

Assuming that patients with slopes lower than the 25th percentile (with steeper slopes), which was -0,0043, are fast progressors and those with slopes higher than the 75th percentile (-0,0006), are slow progressors, we identified 73 patients as low progressors and 53 as fast progressors. Comparisons were made in age, gender, parental origin of the gene, family history of ADPKD, average of the office mean blood pressure (aMBP), number of patients who started dialysis, number of patients who doubled their basal serum creatinine, rate of deterioration of the eGFR, history of gross haematuria, renal colic and urologic manifestations as a whole (Table 1).

As expected, patients belonging to the slow progressors group had lower blood pressure, less episodes of haematuria, less had started dialysis or duplicated basal serum creatinine. Similar results were found if this analysis was restricted to older patients (age over 60 years; data not shown).

Table 1

	Slow progressors	Fast progressors	p
Age	44,5 ± 15,3	49,3 ± 13,2	ns
Sex (M/F)	25/49	16/52	ns
aMBP	100,0 ± 8,3	106,6 ± 8,6	<0,001
decline of eGFR	-1,13 ± 3,35	5,94 ± 2,59	<0,001
Parental origin (F/M)	32/30	12/19	ns
ESRD (y/n)	0/71	30/21	<0,001
Doubling scr (y/n)	0/73	13/40	<0,001
Haematuria (y/n)	15/52	25/17	<0,001
Nephrolithiasis (y/n)	28/39	24/18	ns
Urologic	38/29	33/9	<0,02

Comparisons between slow and fast progression according to the slope of the 1/scr plot (see text for details). Age, in years, refers to the censoring event; aMBP, refers to average office mean blood pressure; decline of eGFR refers to te rate of deterioration of estimated GFR by Cockroft-Gault formula; ESRD, endstage renal disease; doubling scr, refers to the number of patients who doubled their basal serum creatinine during the follow-up; urologic, refers to the number of patients with any urologic symptoms during the follow-up (haematuria, urinary tract infection, cyst infection and renal colic).

Similar results were obtained if categorization was based on the rate of deterioration of renal function evaluated by Cockroft-Gault formula. Fast progressors (52 patients, falling in the 75th percentile or higher [>4,27 ml/min/year]) had a higher aMBP (106,8 ± 6,8 versus 98,6 ± 8,2 mm Hg; p <0,001), started more frequently RRT (27/52 versus 0/51; p<0,001), and doubled basal serum creatinine and had gross haematuria more frequently (doubling scr: 41/52 versus 0/51; p <0,001; haematuria: 23/42 versus 8/46; p< 0,001) than slow progressors (51 patients in the 25th percentile or lower [< 0,17 ml/min/year]).

Discussion

The current study was performed in a large cohort of patients with a long follow-up and the results confirm most of the known risk factors for progression to chronic renal failure. In this study we, like others [12,13], were unable to confirm a gender effect in the progression of ADPKD. Gender is a known risk factor in the progression of diabetic [14] and non-diabetic nephropathy [15-17] and it was also documented in animal models [18-21]. Retrospective studies in ADPKD cohorts gave contradictory results, a few showing no differences between men and women, and some demonstrating a worse prognosis for male [6-8, 22-25]. However, Neugarten [26] published a meta-analysis including 3344 patients with

ADPKD from 12 studies demonstrating a worse renal prognosis for male which is consistent with the finding that male had a faster rate of cyst expansion in the CRISP study [27]. Gender effect is attributed to hormonal influence as the presence of estrogen receptors in mesangial cells may be related to its ability in reducing the rate of collagen production by these cells [28]. The influence of parental origin of the gene was first described by Bear [25] in the population of Newfoundland (Canada) where those who inherited the disease from their mother started RRT earlier than who inherited the disease from their father, an effect designated as imprinting. This effect was attributed to epigenetic effects of DNA modification such as methylation pattern or histone changes that confer greater instability to the genetic material. The effect of imprinting in ADPKD was observed in a few studies [29, 30] but, like us in the current study, not in other [6-9] which is consistent with the fact that, so far, no specific epigenetic modification was described in ADPKD.

Blood pressure is one of the few modifiable risk factors in the ADPKD population. However, the evidence for beneficial effect of lowering blood pressure in the progression of chronic renal failure in this population is mainly indirect [8-31,32]. In the study of Gabow [6] 197 hypertensive patients had a worse renal prognosis than 84 normotensive patients using the 1/scr versus time plot analysis. Similarly, Choukhroun [8] reported an association of the rate of decline of renal function evaluated with Cockroft-Gault formula with mean blood pressure along the follow-up. Few studies evaluated prospectively the effect of anti-hypertensive therapy on the progression of ADPKD. In the MDRD study [33], a separate analysis of the 200 patients with ADPKD revealed disappointed results showing no advantage of strict blood pressure control over usual blood pressure control. However these results were subject of criticism because patients were enrolled in advanced chronic renal disease which could limit the effect of lowering blood pressure. Moreover, attained differences in mean blood pressure were lower than predicted. Likewise, the group of 64 ADPKD patients included in the AIPRI Study [34] also didn't show any retardation of the progression of renal disease. The study of Schrier [35], with a longer follow-up, although showing a beneficial effect on left ventricular mass was, as well, disappointing in what renal protection is concerned.

In our study, office mean blood pressure over a long period of follow-up was used to distinguish patients with good blood pressure control (aMBP <106 mmHg), which had a better renal prognosis, from those with poor control. Office blood pressure is subject to several known influences but serial measurements may reflect the true blood pressure control. In addition to its effect on progression of renal disease, control of hypertension may influence cardiovascular outcomes as we demonstrated in a previous study [38] on this population where the rate of cardiovascular events over the length of follow-up was extremely low.

In the study of Gabow [6] gross haematuria emerged as a risk factor for progression to chronic renal failure but no explanation for this association was provided at that time. However, haematuria as risk factor did not worth further attention of the investigators. In the current study haematuria emerged as one of the most important independent clinical risk factor for progression in ADPKD patients. Although renal volumes were not available in our study we can speculate that haematuria is associated with larger kidney volumes and increasing in renal volume is connected to progression in ADPKD [37]. The influence of other urologic manifestation in renal progression is small in the whole population.

Nevertheless, men who experienced urinary tract infection had a worse prognosis a finding that is in line with those of Gabow [6]. Moreover, combination of urologic symptoms also impose a deleterious effect in men and this fact is an important aspect for those who care for ADPKD patients.

The main limitation of this study is our inability to characterize genetically the population as mutation in PKD1 or PKD2 gene is the most powerful determinant of progression toward RRT in ADPKD patients [7]. Almost all the studies that addressed this question demonstrate that patients bearing PKD1 mutation started RRT considerably earlier than those with PKD2 mutation. The reason for this difference may be related to the finding that in patients with PKD2 phenotype renal cysts appear later and renal volumes are lower than in patients with PKD1 phenotype [38] and this was interpreted as polycystin-1, the product of PKD1 gene, plays an important role in early phases of renal development. However, genetic diagnosis is cumbersome and difficult and not accessible to clinicians which had to provide prognostic information to their patients based mostly on clinical aspects. Other weaknesses of this study are related to the possible effect of referral bias and being an observational uncontrolled rather than interventional and controlled study. However, this study has, in our opinion, a few virtues too. First, this is a longitudinal study done at a single institution where the patients were observed by a single nephrologist for the duration of the follow-up, which reduces the risk for inter-observer variation and also for the practice of nephrology in terms of the most common complications of the disease. Second, the observation time is long (median was 7, up to 29 years of follow-up); third, only few studies have been performed in a population larger than ours [39]. Globally, the results appear to confirm most of the known risk factors for progression in ADPKD patients.

Conclusions

In this longitudinal observational study we provide further support for the evidence that hypertension and haematuria are important risk factors for progression of polycystic kidney disease and may represent important outcomes to achieve in future trials involving ADPKD patients. In summary, in a large cohort of patients with a long time follow-up, the results appear to confirm most of the known risk factors for progression in ADPKD patients.

References

[1] Grantham JJ. Autosomal Dominant Polycystic Kidney Disease. *N. Engl. J .Med.* 2008; 359: 1477-1485.

[2] Torres VE, Harris PC, Pirson Y. Autosomal Dominant Polycystic Kidney Disease. *Lancet* 2007;369:1287-1301.

[3] de Almeida E. Doença Poliquística Renal Autossómica Dominante: Clínica, Genética e Epidemiologia. PhD Thesis. University of Lisbon, 2008.

[4] Ibraghimov-Beskrovnaya O. Molecular pathogenesis of ADPKD and development of targeted therapeutic options. *Nephrol. Dial Transpl* 2007;22:3367-3370.

[5] Hateboer N, van Dijk M, Bogdanova N, Coto E, Saggar-Malik A, San Millan JL, *et al.* Comparison of phenotypes of polycystic kidney disease types 1 and 2. *Lancet* 1999;353:103-107.

[6] Gabow PA, Johnson AM, Kaheny WD, Kimberling WJ, Lezotte DC, Duley IT, *et al.* Factors affecting the progression of renal disease in ADPKD. *Kidney Int.* 1992;41:1311-1319.

[7] Johnson AM, Gabow PA. Identification of patients with ADPKD at highest risk for end-stage renal disease. *J. Am. Soc. Nephrol.* 1997;8:1560-1567.

[8] Choukhroun G, Itakura Y, Albouze G, Christophe JL, Man NK, Grünfeld JP, *et al.* Factors influencing progression of renal failure in ADPKD. *J. Am. Soc. Nephrol.* 1995;6:1634-1642.

[9] Ritz E, Zeier M, Waldherr R. Progression to renal insufficiency. In: Watson ML, Torres VE, ed. *Polycystic kidney disease*. Oxford Medical Publications, Oxford: 1996; 430-449.

[10] Bear JC, McManamon P, Morgan J, Payne RH, Lewis H, Gault MH, *et al.* Age at Clinical onset and at ultrasonographic detection of adult polycystic kidney disease: data for genetic counselling. *Am. J. Med. Genet* 1984;18:45-53.

[11] Cockroft DW, Gault MH. Prediction of creatinine clearance from serum creatinine. *Nephron* 1976; 16:31-41.

[12] Rossetti S, Burton S, Strmecki L, Pond GR, San Millán JL, Zerres K, *et al.* The position of the PKD1 gene mutation correlates with the severity of renal disease. *J. Am. Soc. Nephrol* 2002;13:1230-1237.

[13] Churchill DN, Bear JC, Morgan J, Payne RH, McManamon PJ, Gault MH. Prognosis of adult onset PKD re-evaluated. *Kidney Int* 1984;26:190-193.

[14] West KM, Erdreich LJ, Strober JA. A detailed study of risks factors for retinopathy and nephropathy in diabetes. *Diabetes* 1980;29:501-508.

[15] D'Amico G, Imbasciati E, Barbiano Di Belgioioso G, Bertoli S, Fogazzi G, Ferrario F, *et al.* Idiopathic IgA mesangial nephropathy. Clinical and histological study of 374 patients. *Medicine* (Baltimore) 1985;64:49-60.

[16] Murphy BF, Fairley KF, Kincaid-Smith PS. Idiopathic membranous glomerulonephritis: long-term follow-up in 139 cases. *Clin. Nephrol.* 1988;30:175-181.

[17] Hunt LP, Short CD, Mallick NP. Prognostic indicators in patients presenting with the nephrotic syndrome. *Kidney Int.* 1988;34:382-388.

[18] Kuida S, Beier DR. Genetic localization of interacting modifiers affecting severity in a murine model of PKD. *Genome Res.* 2000;10:49-54.

[19] Remuzzi A, Puntorieri S, Mazzoleni A, Remuzzi G. Sex related differences in ultrafiltration and proteinuria in Munich-Wistar rats. *Kidney Int.* 1988;34:481-486.

[20] Gretz N, Ceccherini I, Kränzlin B, Klötting I, Devotto M, Rohmeiss P, *et al.* Gender-dependent disease severity in autosomal polycystic kidney disease of rats. *Kidney Int* 1995;48:496-500.

[21] Yoshida I, Bengal R, Torres VE. Gender-dependent effect of L-NAME on PKD in Han:SPRD rats. *Am. J. Kidney Dis.* 2000;35:930-936.

[22] Gretz N, Zeier M, Geberth S, Strauch M, Ritz E. Is gender a determinant for evolution of renal failure? A study in Autosomal Dominant Polycystic Kidney Disease. *Am. J. Kidney Dis.* 1989;14:178-183.

[23] Klahr S, Breyer J, Beck GJ, Dennis VW, Hartman JA, Roth D, *et al.* Dietary protein restriction, blood pressure control, and the progression of polycystic kidney disease. *J Am Soc Nephrol* 1995;5:2037-2047.

[24] Torra R, Badenas C, Darnell A, Nicolau C, Volpini V, Revert L, *et al.* Linkage, clinical features, and prognosis of ADPKD types 1 and 2. *J. Am. Soc. Nephrol.* 1996;7:2142-2151.

[25] Bear JC, Parfrey PS, Morgan JM, Martin CJ, Cramer BC. ADPKD: new information for genetic counselling. *Am. J. Med. Genet* 1992;43:548-553.

[26] Neugarten J, Acharya A, Silbiger SR. Effect of gender on the progression of nondiabetic renal disease. *J. Am. Soc. Nephrol.* 2000;11:319-329.

[27] Harris PC, Bae KT, Rossetti S, Torres VE, Grantham JJ, Chapman AB, e tal. Cyst number but not the rate of cystic growth is associated with the mutated gene in Autosomal Dominant Polycystic Kidney Disease. *J. Am. Soc. Nephrol.* 17; 3013-3019, 2006.

[28] Kwan G, Neugarten J, Sherman M, Ding Q, Fotadar U, Lei J, *et al.* Effects of sex hormones on mesangial cell proliferation and collagen synthesis. *Kidney Int.* 1996;50:1173-1179.

[29] Fick GM, Johnson AM, Gabow PA. Is there evidence for antecipation in ADPKD? *Kidney Int* 1994;45:1153-1162.

[30] Zerres K, Rudnik-Schöneborn S, Deget F. Childhood onset ADPKD in sibs: clinical picture and recurrence risk. *J. Med. Genet* 1993;30:583-588.

[31] Geberth S, Stier E, Mayer G, Rambausek M, Ritz E. More adverse renal prognosis of ADPKD in families with primary hypertension. *J. Am. Soc. Nephrol.* 1995;6:1643-1648.

[32] Schrier RW, Johnson AM, McFann K, Chapman A. The role of parental hypertension in the frequency and age of diagnosis of hypertension in offsprig with ADPKD. *Kidney Int* 2003;64:1792-1799.

[33] Klahr S, Breyer J, Beck GJ, Dennis VW, Hartman JA, Roth D, *et al.* Dietary protein restriction, blood pressure control, and the progression of polycystic kidney disease. *J. Am. Soc. Nephrol.* 1995;5:2037-2047.

[34] Maschio G, Alberti D, Janin G, Locatelli F, Mann J, Motolese M, *et al.* Effect of the Angiotensin Converting Enzyme inhibitor benazepril on the progression of chronic renal insufficiency. *N. Engl. J. Med.* 1996;334:939-945.

[35] Schrier RW, McFann K, Johnson AM, Chapman A, Edelstein C, Brosnahan G, *et al.* Cardiac and Renal Effects of Standard versus Rigorous Blood Pressure Control in ADPKD: results of a seven-year prospective randomized study. *J. Am. Soc. Nephrol.* 2002;13:1733-1739.

[36] de Almeida E, Prata MM. Hipertensão arterial na doença poliquística renal autossómica dominante: estudo observacional em 207 doentes com follow-up médio de 107 meses. *Rev. Port Cardiol.* 2007; 26: 1173-1182.

[37] Grantham JJ, Torres VE, Chapman AB, Guay-Woodford LM, Bae KT, King BF, *et al.* Volume progression in polycystic kidney disease. *N. Engl. J. Med.* 2006;354:2122-2130.

[38] Harris PC, Bae KT, Rossetti S, Torres VE, Grantham JJ, Chapman AB, *et al.* Cyst number but not the rate of cyst growth is associated with the mutated gene in Autosomal Dominant Polycystic Kidney Disease. *J. Am. Soc. Nephrol.* 2006; 17:3013-3019.

[39] Schrier RW, Mc Fann KK, Johnson AM. Epidemiological study of kidney survival in autosomal dominant polycystic kidney disease. *Kidney Int.* 2003; 63: 678-685.

In: Nephrology – Dialysis - Transplantation
Editors: Endre Kruger and Kelemen Hahn

ISBN 978-1-60741-736-1
© 2009 Nova Science Publishers, Inc.

Chapter VII

Genetics in Clinical Nephrology

Hansjörg Rothe
Kuratorium für Dialyse and Nierentransplantation,
Dept. of Nephrology and Hypertension, Klinikum Neumarkt, Germany

1. Population Genetics

1.1. Epidemiology of Chronic Kidney Disease

Chronic kidney disease (CKD) often clusters within families. Studies have suggested possible links between CKD and a variety of alterations or polymorphisms of candidate genes coding for putative mediators, including the renin angiotensin aldosterone system (RAAS), nitric oxide synthetase, kallikrein, interleukin 1, tumour necrosis factor α and other cytokines, growth factors such as platelet derived growth factor and transforming growth factor β, plasminogen activator inhibitor, complement factors and immunoglobulins [1].

Nevertheless there seems to be a fairly stable proportion of people throughout the world regardless of their genetic background who show signs of early stage CKD, although the distributions of etiology (incidence of diabetes, pyelonephritis, Mediterranean fever etc.) differ. In the United States, Japan, the United Kingdom, Germany, the Netherlands and Australia epidemiological surveys showed a constant estimate of 9-12% of people between 25 and 80 years with proteinuria, albuminuria and/or decreased kidney function.

1.2. Epidemiology of Diabetic Nephropathy

On the one hand, only between 30–40% with diabetes type I and 10–20% of type II diabetics will develop nephropathy. On the other hand nephropathy may develop in some patients despite excellent blood sugar control, but it may fail to develop in others despite long-term hyperglycemia. Clinically one can apply the rule that the presence of retinopathy makes it more likely that nephropathy will also develop, whereas in patients who have had a history of 20 years of diabetes without renal involvement the occurrence of significant diabetic nephropathy is unlikely. These findings suggest that apart from the actual blood sugar control there are hereditary and environmental factors contributing to the development of diabetic nephropathy [2]. The prevalence of nephropathy among diabetics is variable in different ethnic groups such that it is relatively increased in African Americans, Native Americans, Mexican Americans, Polynesians, Australian Aborigines and urbanized Indo-Asian immigrants to the United Kingdom when compared to Caucasians. Apart from the genetic make-up, social factors such as the accessibility of health care certainly play a role in some of these populations.

Familial clustering of diabetic nephropathy (DN) has been reported in both type I and type II diabetes and in both Caucasian and non-Caucasian populations. In a type I diabetic with a first degree relative who has diabetes and nephropathy, the risk of developing DN is 83%, but it drops to 17% if the first degree relative has diabetes but no nephropathy. In the Native American Pima population familial clustering has been well documented for type II diabetes. The risk for children to later develop nephropathy is particularly high if the mother had been hyperglycemic during pregnancy, presumably this leads to reduced nephron formation ("nephron underdosing"), as shown in animal models. Gene polymorphisms may also play a role in familial clustering. Candidate polymorphisms for associations with predisposition to DN are in the carnosinase gene (leading to cumulation of carnosine with antioxidant properties) and a double delete polymorphism of the angiotensin converting enzyme gene which leads to accelerated progression of DN.

1.3. Epidemiology of Arterial Hypertension

In the development of arterial hypertension the influence of nutritional and environmental factors is paramount, as illustrated by the results of the Intersalt study [3]. Disease progression correlates positively with weight gain, alcohol consumption, and to some degree salt intake.

There are genetic factors involved though, which is obvious looking at familial clustering, 70% of hypertensive patients have a positive family history [4]. Monozygotic twins will more often have parallel development of hypertension as compared with heterozygote twins. There are genetically defined populations with significantly increased hypertension incidence, such as Afro-Americans in the US. Investigations in patients with essential hypertension showed links to various candidate genes, such as angiotensinogen, adducin (which is part of the cytoskeleton and involved in salt reabsorption), the beta-adrenergous receptor and several other genes coding for subunits of the epithelial sodium channel (ENaC).

Some genetic tubular disorders (see 4.) are also associated with hypertension.

2. Pharmacogenetics

2.1. Introduction - Concept of Pharmacogenetics

Hippocrates is believed to have coined the sentence: It is more important to know *who* has a disease, than to know what disease someone has. That shows that pharmacotherapy being as individualized as possible has been regarded as an ideal since ancient times—especially since "the dosage makes the poison", as Paracelsus pointed out, i.e. adverse effects can easily obscure the healing success. With some justification the concept of pharmacogenetics may be described as the scientific quintessence of these two ancient medical sayings: the individual response to any medicine is influenced by the genetic makeup of the patient which therefore should be taken into consideration before dosing.

In principle, genetic factors can interfere in two ways with pharmacotherapy— with pharmacokinetics (i.e. achieving sufficient concentrations of the active compound at the site of action) and with pharmacodynamics (i.e. the interaction of the active compound with its receptor). An example for the former is the cytochrome P450 enzymes, or the MDR1/ABCB1 gene product, a transport protein which forms an absorption barrier by carrying various compounds back into the intestinal lumen (efflux pump, related to the SLC uptake transporter). Examples for the latter would be the polymorphisms of the calcimimetic receptor and the angiotensin receptors.

Even though the term "pharmacogenetics" is relatively old, we have only started to move towards clinical practicability in recent years. Reinhard J. Haschen gave the headline "overdosing, pharmacogenetics" to one of the chapters in his textbook "Enzymdiagnostik" (enzyme diagnostics) in 1968, in this chapter he discussed the genetic variants of choline esterase, which lead to different metabolism and therefore activity of succinyldicholin and other muscle relaxants. Some phenotypic tests such as the ABO blood group system and HLA antigens have been in use for several decades. Meanwhile we know that apart from isoenzymes—i.e. variants of an enzyme which is expressed slightly differently in organs or individuals—there are similar variants in receptors, too, which are referred to as "isoreceptors" accordingly. The basis of this variability is polymorphism on the DNA level; some of these polymorphisms are arranged in clusters and cause ethnic variability or "races" that way. Individual differences in the metabolism of pharmaca can be brought about by polymorphisms of enzymes such as cytochrome P450 enzymes or transport proteins such as MDR efflux pumps.

Today there is already a number of obligatory pharmacogenetic tests in some medical specialities: Prior to a therapy of breast cancer with trastuzumab, a genetic test concerning epidermal growth factor receptor HER2 has to be performed, the two main methods used for HER2 testing are immunohistochemistry (IHC) and fluorescence in-situ hybridization (FISH) Another example is the HLA-B*5701 test in HIV therapy with abacavir. In this chapter, areas of nephrological practice will be discussed, where pharmacogenetic methods can already be utilized with benefit.

2.2. Calcineurin inhibitors

Pharmacotherapy with potentially toxic substances can be monitored either with the blood level of the drug, or by measurement of a parameter showing the toxic effect. Calcineurin inhibitors are widely used for maintenance immunosuppression after kidney transplantation, and the standard procedure to prevent calcineurin inhibitor nephrotoxicity is blood level monitoring of the drug. Recent findings provide first evidence that ABCB1 genetics may be of clinical relevance for treatment of kidney recipients with cyclosporine, which is one member of the calcineurin inhibitor family. [5,6] It is the genotype of the donor, not of the recipient, which is important here – if the transmembrane efflux pump P-glycoprotein expression is reduced in the transplanted organ because of an ABCB1 polymorphism, lower blood levels of the drug have to be aimed for in order to prevent toxic levels within the kidney.

2.3. Azathioprine

Unlike calcineurin inhibitor therapy (see above), the treatment with potentially myelosuppressive azathioprine is not monitored by checking the blood levels of the drug, but the white cell counts. Pharmacogenetic gold standard as a method to reduce the amounts of necessary white cell counts used to be the measurement of TPMT activity until recently. This highly polymorphic enzyme determines the speed of azathioprine metabolism and excretion, measuring its activity helps for dose stratification, reduction of toxic complications, and saving costs [7]. Since an excellent phenotype-genotype correlation does exist and several high-throughput genotyping methods are available, azathioprine is actually another example where performing a pharmacogenetic test is proven to be clinically useful. [8,9]. This test needs to be performed only once, white cell counts are necessary less often, for fine tuning of the dose. The therapeutic level is reached faster, with fewer adverse effects, which all together reduces costs. Interestingly, there are remarkable differences between specialists in how often they use the test for azathioprine dosing. British dermatologists test almost always, gastroenterologists and rheumatologists far less often [10]. To come to a consensus, a randomized controlled trial has been performed in the British health service (TARGET) which is already closed, the results are not published yet .

2.4. Vitamin-K Antagonists and Thrombocyte Aggregation Inhibitors

Coumarines and antiplatelet drugs such as clopidogrel are used quite often in nephrology, the latter not only for cardiovascular protection but also to prevent shunt thrombosis in patients on maintenance hemodialysis. Because of several factors interfering with coagulation and platelet function in nephrological patients, dosing and monitoring is especially difficult, though. Recently a pharmacogenetic test for polymorphisms of VCORC1 and CYP2C9 genes, which are relevant for coumarine metabolism, was recommended by the US Food and

Drug Administration [11]. Another influential cytochrome is CYP4F2 [12]. These tests again need to be performed only once and allow for dose stratification, faster achievement of target range with fewer clotting tests. However, clinical or phenotypic factors as well as genetic ones need to be considered. Washington University Medical Center have developed a tool based on both types of evidence and offer it a free website (www.warfarindosing.org). Considering high costs of hospitalization because of coumarine side effects world wide this test is interesting from a health economics perspective, too [13]. It has already been proven in prospective trials that a genotype-guided approach is superior to standard warfarin dosing [14,15]. The best strategy for a stable anticoagulation from the beginning seems to be a pharmacogenetically stratified starting dose with subsequent administration of coumarine together with a small dose of vitamin K which diminishes diet-induced changes of blood vitamin K levels [16]. Most studies in this area were performed with warfarin, similar investigations are needed for phenprocoumon.

Platelet response to the ADP receptor blocker clopidogrel is heavily influenced by the polymorphism of CYP2C19 [17]. Since protein pump inhibitors such as omeprazole are metabolised by the same enzyme, co-administration with clopidogrel can lead to inactivation of the latter and has to be avoided.

2.5. Calcimimetics

Since its FDA approval in 2004 Cinacalcet HCL has become a major therapy option for secondary, primary and persisting post-transplant hyperparathyroidism as well as parathyroid carcinoma. In patients with chronic kidney disease the connection between the parathyroid hormone/calcium/phosphate problem, especially adynamic bone disease, and cardiovascular mortality is better understood in recent years ("Treat the bone to keep the vessels clear"). Response rates to cinacalcet were satisfactory in all clinical studies so far; on average a PTH suppression of at least 30–40% could be achieved with a decrease of calcium and phosphate at the same time. We investigated genetic polymorphisms (see figure 1) of the calcium-sensing receptor as one possible explanation for interindividual variability in dose response [18]. Three such polymorphisms — $Arg^{990}Gly$, $Ala^{986}Ser$ and $Glu^{1011}Gln$[1] — were described in exon 7 of the receptor gene, which encodes the C-terminal intracellular end of the molecule (see figure 2). All three of them are single nucleotide polymorphisms (SNP), since only one nucleotide is variable.

Some papers point to a clinical significance of at least one of these three SNP's : a Japanese group investigated PTH suppression after a mild hypercalcemic stimulus in 77 hemadialysis patients. They found that 5 patients with arginine in position 990 had no PTH suppression after a defined stimulus which was sufficient to cause PTH suppression in 33 patients with glycine in the same position as well as 39 heterozygous patients [19].

A dose response study with 23 hemodialysis patients found an influence of polymorphism Arg990Gly on PTH suppression after the administration of a single dose of

---

[1] In this way of referring to polymorphisms the more frequent allele comes first, in the middle the number of the amino acid starting from the N-terminus, at the end the less frequent allele.

60mg cinacalcet [20]. Patients with at least one glycine allele achieved significantly more often a PTH suppression by at least 5% after 24h as compared with the group of arginine homozygotes, which predominates in Blacks and Whites (odds ratio 2,6). (see Figure 3).

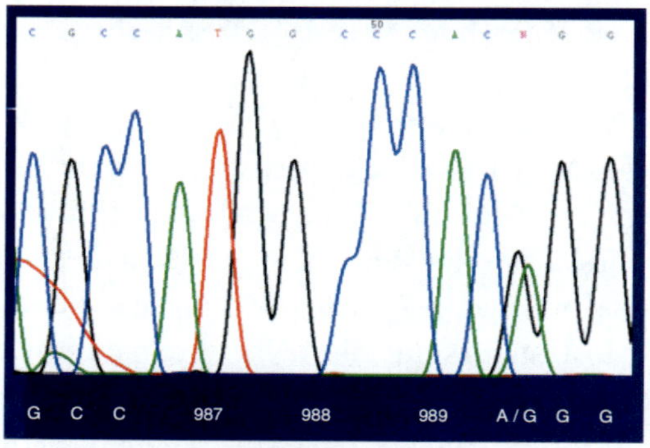

Figure 1. Example for a nucleotide sequence: Patient heterozygous in position 990.

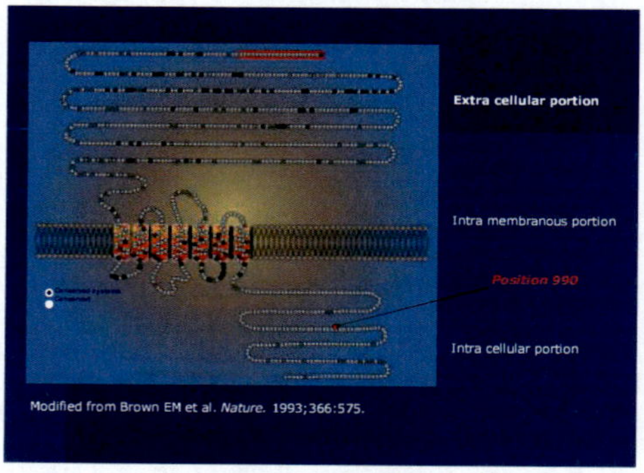

Figure 2. position 990 of the calcium-sensitive receptor as an example of a polymorphic site

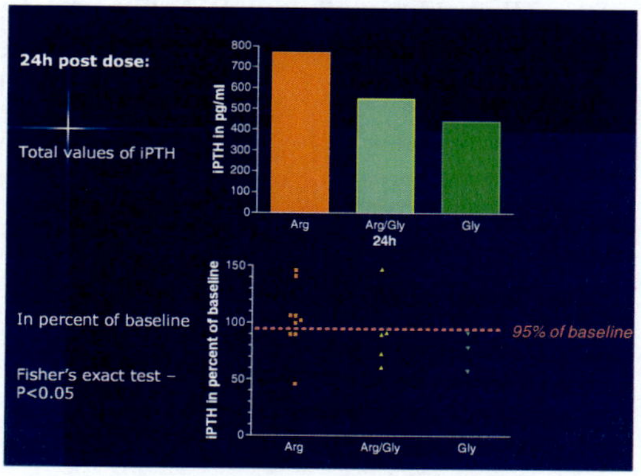

Figure 3. PTH suppression at 24h after a single dose of 60mg Cinacalcet

In an Austrian epidemiological study with 82 Caucasian hemodialysis patients, there were 10% patients with one glycine allele. In these patients one would expect better response to lower doses, but also stronger side effects in cases of overdosing. Asian patients on the other hand have almost always (95%) at least one glycine allele, and that explains why they need even lower doses than their body mass would suggest.

Causal relationship for this polymorphism Arg990Gly could be demonstrated in cell culture by transfection of human embryonic kidney cells with the two different isoforms of the receptor [21]. It needs to be clarified in a clinical trial, in which patients it would make sense to do the pharmacogenetic test in order to improve calcimimetic therapy.

2.6. Opioid Derivatives

In kidney disease patients, renal elimination is decreased or totally absent. Polymorphisms of cytochrome P450 enzymes affecting hepatic clearance of toxic substances may become clinically important even without renal failure but especially under these circumstances, which can be illustrated by the danger of opioid accumulation. Especially CYP2D6 is important here because of several activating and inactivating variants of this enzyme, due to genetic polymorphism [22]. In a tragic case a newborn died in Canada in 2006 after the mother had been given codeine for pain relief — even though she had no kidney failure, her Cytochrome P2D6 polymorphism, leading to ultrarapid metabolism of codeine to morphine, was sufficient to cause extremely high morphine concentrations in the milk and a fatal intoxication of the child [23]. If there is clinical suspicion of a cytochrome P450 polymorphism this can be tested with a genotyping test, several chips specialising in this class of enzymes are available on the market.

2.7. Cardiovascular Protective Therapy

For many years polymorphisms of the renin angiotensin aldosterone system have been studied. Genetic influence on this hugely important pathway is well documented, for instance Black patients are known to show very little reponse to the same drugs interfering in the RAAS system that are successfully used in Asian or Caucasian subjects. However so far there are only few hard data with clinical siginificance: As far as angiotensin converting enzyme (ACE) is concerned, plasma and tissue levels of ACE are at least partially determined by a genetic polymorphism based on the presence (insertion, I) or absence (deletion, D) of a 287 base pair element in intron 16. It has been reported that in particular Asian subjects with the DD genotype (and increased ACE activity) are at higher risk for cardiovascular disorders and nephropathy. Several studies evaluated the role of the ACE I/D polymorphism as well as other genetic variants of the RAAS in the context of RAAS inhibitor therapy. However, as race and environmental factors like salt intake also affect treatment response most studies were underpowered leading to conflicting results.

Apart from the RAAS system, there are several potentially interesting findings for other drugs of cardiovascular protective therapy. For instance some haplotype blocks in the gene of endothelial NO synthetase are associated with an increased risk of hypertension in pregnancy and preeclampsia [24]. Patients who will benefit from a heart failure therapy with bucindolol may be identified with a pharmacogenetic test for polymorphisms of their endothelin 1 gene, also a subgroup that will tend to get negative outcomes from bucindolol [25]. Bucindolol is therefore an example for a promising compound which was withdrawn from the market because of a randomized controlled trial but could be "rescued" by pharmacogenetic tests, allowing us to sort out which patients will benefit from the drug and which won't (this would be desirable for COX-2 inhibitors or cervistatin, too, among others).

Regarding both pharmacokinetic and pharmacodynamic influence of polymorphisms (P.) on statin therapy there have been several reports about association of polymorphisms with various phenotypes in certain populations. This problem can serve as an example for the difficult task of interpreting such association in a complex intercation of several genes and pathways. There have been papers published about HindIII P. of lipoproteine lipase [26], the CYP2D6*4 P. [27], the A1166C P. of the AT1 receptor gene [28], the C-107T P. of the paraoxonase 1 gene promoter [29], the -514C/T P. of the hepatic lipase gene [30] and the TaqIB P. in the CETP gene [31], however the question of potential clinical relevance hasn't been solved so far in all these cases. In fact most of them have not been confirmed by independent studies. In contrast a prominent top candidate gene related to the most important adverse effect of statin therapy – statin induced myopathy – could be identified by the SEARCH collaborative group in a genome wide association study [32].

There is no doubt that vitamin D therapy may be associated with an increased risk of developing soft tissue and arterial calcification. However, any hopes for a pharmacogenetic test to select high and low risk patients haven't been fulfilled so far. In one report about a Spanish patient cohort a strong correlation between a vitamin D receptor gene polymorphism (BsmI) and cardiovascular mortality was detected, but in a German study 3441 patients who had coronary angiography performed didn't show any association between polymorphism status and signs of coronary artery disease [33]. In general it needs to be stressed that singular findings of association between a polymorphic allele and a phenotypic symptom doesn't necessarily mean that there must be a causal relation, since polymorphisms are arranged in haplotype blocks quite often, as mentioned earlier. The suspected effect might be connected with a totally different gene, and in other populations different haplotype arrangements might be prevalent.

2.8. Outlook

In contrast to cardiology, randomised controlled multi-center trials did not produce a lot of hard reliable mortality reduction data in nephrology, despite various efforts in recent decades [34]. Insiders expect that the wording of this year's KDIGO initiative recommendations, which are based on these hard data, will be less strict as compared with the older KDOQI guidelines, leaving more room for interpretation [35]. It seems that the global multi-center approach is not the optimal tool to depict nephrological hypotheses. One reason might be that with increasing complexity of causal relations involved, the specific polymorphism clusters of a given population become more relevant. Conceivably new impulses could come in the future from a more individualized abstraction as opposed to a merely generalising abstraction — as a concept of science metatheory this approach was developed already by Max Weber in the early 20th century, maybe now with our new knowledge of genetics and individualized medicine the time has come for this concept to bear fruit. With smaller patient numbers, but exact definition of the genetic make-up of the patient groups, effects may be depictable that otherwise had gone unnoticed in a large but ill defined pool. For instance, carriers of certain alleles of the SGK1 gene are largely protected against the development of diabetes type II [36] — if patient cohorts from different populations with different prevalence of these alleles are lumped together with the intention of studying proteinuria, one might achieve big patient numbers, but no decent results. Retrospective investigations, such as one that was recently started about the influence of CYP3A5 polymorphisms on tacrolimus based immunosuppression after life kidney transplants, provide hypotheses for prospective studies. Time will show if vitamin D receptor polymorphisms can play a role in clinical decisions about vitamin D therapy. The fact that some patients despite long-term steroid therapy never develop osteoporosis, may be due to genetic isoforms of the glucocorticoid receptor and might be useful for pharmacogenetics in the future. Similarly, testing for polymorphisms of catechol-O-methyltransferase (COMT), which also plays a role in depression, might become a tool to predict the risk of acute renal failure after cardiac surgery due to noradrelanine resistance [37].

3. Genetics of Polycystic Kidney Disease

3.1. Autosomal Dominant Polycystic Kidney Disease

In 85–90% of clinically detected cases of ADPKD, the PKD1 gene is responsible. Most other patients show abnormalities of the PKD2 gene on chromosome 4, but a third gene may exist, as evidenced by absence of linkage with either PKD1 or PKD2 in some families [38].

There is also an independent clinical entity characterized by liver cysts without renal involvement. This syndrome called autosomal dominant polycystic liver disease is genetically heterogenous, two genes were identified so far (PRKCSH in chromosome 19 and Sec63 in chromosome 6). The fact that only a small percentage of nephrons will develop cysts in ADPKD gave rise to a theory of two-hit etiology of cystogenesis similar to the tumor suppressor model in carcinogenesis. Loss of heterozygosity with deletion of a wild type PKD gene can be demonstrated in 30% of cysts, which arise from clonal expansion of a single cell. Mice with single PKD1 or PKD2 copies have only a mild phenotype, whereas homozygous pkd1 or pkd2 null mouse embryos have severe cystic changes. On the other hand, pkd1 overexpression and aberrant splicing will also lead to cyst formation.

The proteins encoded by the PKD genes are called polycystin 1 and 2; they play an important role in intracellular calcium homeostasis. The extracellular portion of polycystin 1 has some homology to proteins involved in sperm-egg interaction and the acrosome reaction. Polycystin 2 is basically a calcium permeable cation channel. Both proteins do activate a number of intracellular pathways (G protein, Wnt, JAK/STAT signalling).

The polycystin complex is present in primary cilia; it mediates calcium fluxes as a response to mechanical stimulation. Primary cilia are hair-like cell organelles arising from the centrosome, which is the microtubule organizing centre of the cell; they project from the surface of most mammalian cells. Disruption of the primary cilia in the principal cells of collecting ducts leads to a phenotype of polycystic kidney disease.

Prognosis of ADPKD is mainly dependent on which gene is affected. PKD1 genotype, male gender and onset before age 30 are poor prognosis markers. The disease is less common in Blacks than in Whites and affects between 1:400 and 1:1000 individuals. It does occur worldwide, but less often in Africa.

Two promising therapeutic options for slowing down the growth of the cysts have been tested so far in clinical trials: everolimus and tolvaptane. Final analysis of the trial results are not yet available, but expected to be published within the next year.

3.2. Other Cystic Kidney Diseases

Apart from ADPKD there are other genetic disorders which appear with similar clinical pictures of renal cystic disease: von Hippel Lindau syndrome, Tuberous sclerosis, adult-onset medullary cystic disease, autosomal recessive polycystic kidney disease, Meckel-Gruber-Syndrome, juvenile nephronophtisis and the X-linked orafaciodigital syndrome type 1.

Von Hippel Lindau Syndrome is dominantly transmitted, predisposing to malignancies in various organ systems including the nervous system, pancreas, adrenal glands, epididymis as well as pancreatic and renal cysts. It is caused by mutations in the VHL tumor suppressor gene on chromosome 3. In 80% of cases, it is familial, in the rest of the cases spontaneous. Up to 75% of VHL patients will develop renal cell carcinoma by age 60.

The physiological role of the VHL protein lies in oxygen sensing. It downregulates several members of the hypoxia-inducible factor (HIF) family by marking them for degradation via the ubiquitine pathway.

Tuberous sclerosis is characterized by angiomyolipomas or hamartomas in the nervous system, the skin (adenoma sebaceum), the kidneys, the lungs or other organs. Together with von Hippel Lindau disease it is referred to as phakomatosis, underlying mutations affect the TSC1 and 2 genes.

4. Genetic Tubular Syndromes

4.1. Proximal Tubule Disorders

There is a genetic variant of Fanconi's syndrome. This condition is autosomal dominant and localized on chromosome 15. The clinical picture begins with lactaciduria and proteinuria in early childhood, later glucosuria and aminoaciduria develop in the 2nd decade of life. Later osteomalacia occurs from the 4th decade.

For secondary Fanconi's due to cystinosis see 7.

4.2. Tubular Syndromes Associated with Hypotension

The clinical condition of Bartter's syndrome (polyuria, polydipsia, tendency to dehydration, salt loss with hypokalemia and hypomagnesemia, sometimes nephrocalcinosis) can be divided into 5 different genotypes. In Type 1, also referred to as antenatal Bartter's syndrome (BS) type I or hyperprostaglandin E syndrome, the Na-K-2Cl cotransporter is affected. This defect is localized on gene SLC12A1 and leads to a picture similar to continous furosemide infusion.

Type 2 or antenatal BS type II is due to inactivating mutations of the ROMK gene (ATP sensitive potassium channel)

Type 3 is the classical BS, which accounts for 60% of cases. The basolateral chloride channel in Henle's loop is dysfunctional.

In type 4 there is deafness in addition to renal symptoms, since a protein is affected, which forms heteromeres with chloride channels and is present in the inner ear lymph forming epithelia in addition to Henle's loop.

Type 5 BS is similar to type 2 in that the ROMK is dysfunctional, however this is caused by inhibition of otherwise normal ROMK due to activating mutations of the calcium-sensing receptor which leads to profound hypocalcemia in addition to other Bartter symptoms.

Gitelman's syndrome is a condition of the distal tubule. The thiazide-sensitive Na-K-Cl cotransporter is inactivated leading to salt loss, cramps and muscle weakness. 45% of patients describe their condition as a moderate health problem.

Genetic variants of nephrogenic diabetes insipidus are mostly X-linked and affect the vasopressin 2 receptor in the collecting ducts, which gets degraded faster and is less efficient in the binding of vasopressin (antidiuretic hormone). There is also an autosomal recessive type which affects ADH sensitive aquaporine 2. In rare cases Fabry's disease can cause nephrogenic diabetes insipidus (see 7.)

4.3. Tubular Syndromes Associated With Hypertension

There are several autosomal dominant syndromes associated with hypertension due to single gene mutations: glucocorticoid-sensitive hyperaldosteronism is caused by a gene chimera between the two genes for aldosteronsynthetase and 11-β-Hydroxylase. The gene has the promoter of 11-β-hydroxylase, is therefore activated by ACTH and produces aldosterone in the adrenal gland's zona fasciculata. Clinically, hypertension in these patients disappears with 5mg prednisone per day. Since it was first described by Lifton more then 100 families have been identified worldwide.

Liddle syndrome is also salt-sensitive, but hypertension doesn't respond to spironolactone, but to amiloride and triamterene. Mutations in one of the subunits of the ENaC lead to an overactive sodium and chloride reabsorption in the collecting ducts.

S810L mutation of the mineralocorticoid receptor leads to a hyperactivity of the receptor and to its activation by spironolactone and progesterone. Pregnant women with the mutation will therefore develop hypertensive crises.

Gordon Syndrome is also called pseudohypoaldosteronism type 2. It is caused by mutations in either of two serine-threonine kinases called WNK1 and WNK4. These kinases ("with no lysine", therefore WNK) are involved in the regulation of the thiazide-sensitive sodium-chloride cotransporter, hypertenison in these patients responds to thiazide.

Hypertension with brachydaktyly occurs in patients with a mutation on chromosome 12p.

There is a syndrome characterized by hypertension, hyperlipidemia, hypokalemia and hypomagnesemia which is due to the mutation in a gene of the mitochondrial DNA.

Apparent mineralocorticoid excess is autosomal recessive. It can be mimicked by excessive intake of lacorice, since this contains inhibitor substances of 11 β dehydroxygenase. In the syndrome cortisole is not degraded to cortisone in the distal tubulus and activates the mineralocorticoid receptor continuously, leading to hyperreabsorption of sodium and chloride.

About 30% of patients with pheochromozytoma in Europe develop this condition because of a genetic defect, such as von Hippel Lindau syndrome, MEN 2 syndrome, neurofibromatosis type I or either of two mutations in a subunit of succinyldehydrogenase.

5. Genetic Glomerular Syndromes

Alport's syndrome is caused by a lack of type IV collagen, leading to dysfunctional glomerular basal membranes. Mutations affecting subunits COL4A3, COL4A4 or COL4A5 will all result in the same weak membranes made up only of embruonal collagen α1 and α2 chains. Extrarenal symptoms typically involve inner ear deafness, but the eye (retina , lens) can also be affected, as well as platelets (impaired platelet function). The classical genetic background is X-linked, but there are also autosomal recessive variants.

Recessive forms of the disease without the full clinical picture are referred to as thin Basement membrane nephropathy.

Nail Patella Syndrome is also associated with a defect of collagen IV, due to a mutation of the LMX1B gene.

There is a number of congenital nephrotic syndromes. All of them are autosomal. In the so-called Finnish type a protein called nephrin is knocked out, which is essential for podocyte function. A steroid-resistant type is caused by a mutation in the NPHS2/SRNS gene coding for podocine, another podocyte protein. Congenital focal segmental glomerular sclerosis is brought about by mutations in FSG2 or FSG3 genes. Denys-Drash-syndrome is a diffuse mesangial sclerosis caused by mutation of the WT1/DMS gene.

6. Genetic Background of Sickle Cell Disease

Originating from West Africa, where it may have been associated with a survival benefit due to malaria, this autosomal recessive single nucleotide mutation has now spread all over the world. The highest prevalence in the US is among African Americans, but in some areas in the Mediterranean and Middle East up to 25% of people carry the hemoglobin S allele. In hemoglobin S conformational changes are caused by a replacement of a single amino acid (glutamine by valine). Patients develop impaired concentrating capacity quite early, hematuria associated with glomerular pathology such as FSGS and papillary necroses later and chronic renal failure in about 5% of patients with sickle cell anemia and 2.5% in those with sickle cell trait.

7. Genetic Metabolic Disorders

Fabry's disease is also referred to as angiokeratoma corporis diffusum and is caused by defects in the lysosomal α-galactosidase gene. The result of a lack of the enzyme is accumulation of glycosphingolipids in lysosomes and endothelium mainly in kidneys, the heart, skin and nervous system. Cerebrovascual accidents in young adults are often due to undiagnosed Fabry's.

In the kidneys early symptoms are a mild proteinuria and hematuria. From the 2nd to 4th decade progressive renal failure and secondary arterial hypertension will occur if untreated (intravenous substitution of α-galactosidase every 4–6 weeks).

Cystinosis is autosomal recessive and is caused by mutations in a lysosomal protein which is necessry for the transport of the amino acid cystin from lysosomes into the cytosol. Lack of this protein leads to accumulation of cystin within the lysosomes and results in proximal tubular damage with Fanconi's syndrome, osteomalcia due to phosphate loss, renal tubular acidosis, and often end-stage kidney disease in childhood. There is an intermediate variant and the adult type, in which patients are mostly asymptomatic apart from cystin cristall deposition in the corneae.

Genetic reasons for the hyperoxaluria syndrome are two enzyme defects leading to oxalate cumulation. Both defects are autosomal recessive. Patients present with recurrent gall bladder and or kidney stones. In 50% of patients symptoms will occur before the age of five, 50% of patients will develop end-stage kidney disease by age 15. [39].

Acknowledgments

Many thanks for advise and suggestions to Prof. Gert Mayer, University of Innsbruck (Austria), and Dr. Joanne Blanchfield, University of Queensland (Australia).

References

[1] Mohsen el Kossi and Meguid el Nahas in *Comprehensive clinical nephrology*, p.813 , Feehally Floege and Johnson, Philadelphia 2007.

[2] Eberhard Ritz in *Comprehensive clinical nephrology*, p. 357 , Feehally Floege and Johnson, Philadelphia 2007. *BMJ* 1988, 297(6644):319-28.

[3] F.C.Luft in *Nephrologie*, p.490 – 6, Kuhlmann, Walb, Böhler and Luft, Stuttgart/New York 2008.

[4] Eichelbaum M et al. *Ther Drug Monit.* 26:180-5, 2004.

[5] Hauser IA et al., *JASN* 16 :1501-1511, 2005
[6] Cattaneo et al., *JASN* 20 :1404-1415, 2009
[7] Fargher EA et al. *J. Clin. Pharm. Ther.* 32:187-95, 2007.
[8] Sahasranaman et al., *Eur J Clin Pharmacol* 64:753-767, 2008
[9] Teml A et al., *Clin Phramacokinet* 46:187-208, 2007
[10] Payne K *Rheumatology (Oxford)* 46 :727-9, 2007
[11] Thompson C. *Am. J. Health Syst. Pharm.* 64:1994-6., 2007.
[12] Caldwell M et al *Blood* 111:4106-12, 2008
[13] Eckman MH et al., *Ann Intern Med* 150:73-87, 2009
[14] Anderson JL et al. *Circulation* 116:2563-70, 2007
[15] Caraco Y et al. *Clin Pharmacol Ther* 83:460-70. 2008
[16] Oldenburg J. *Thromb Haemost.* 98:570-8, 2007.
[17] Varenhorst C et al. *Eur Heart J* 30:1744-52, 2009
[18] Rothe H et al. *Pharmacogenet Genomics*. 15:29-34, 2005.
[19] Yokoyama K et al. *Clin. Nephrol.* 57:131–135, 2002.
[20] Rothe H et al. *Personalized Medicine* 5:109-116, 2008.
[21] Vezzoli G et al. *Kidney Int.* 71:1155-62, 2007.
[22] Koren G et al. *Lancet* 19:704
[23] Madadi P et al. *Can. Fam. Physician.* 53:33-5, 2007.
[24] Sandrim VC et al. *Pharmacogenomics* 9:1467-73, 2008.
[25] Taylor MR et al. *Pharmacogenet Genomics* Epub ahead of print, 2008.
[26] Javorsky M et al. *Wien Klin Wochenschr.* 119:476-82, 2007.
[27] Frudakis TN et al. *Pharmacogenet Genomics*. 17:695-707, 2007.
[28] Kiliszek M et al. *Clin. Chem. Lab. Med.* 45:839-42, 2007.
[29] Deakin Set al. *Pharmacogenet Genomics.* 17:451-7, 2007.
[30] Lahoz C et al. *Atherosclerosis.* 182:129-34, 2005.
[31] Mohrschladt MFet al. *Eur. J. Hum. Genet.* 13:877-82, 2005.
[32] Link E *N Engl J Med* 21:789-99, 2008
[33] Ortlepp JR et al. *Eur. J. Clin. Invest.* Feb;33(2):106-9, 2003.
[34] Strippoli GF. *JASN* 15:506-508, 2004.
[35] oral presentation by T. Drueke, 2. IFMO Dresden 15.11.2008.
[36] Schwab M et al. *Cell Physiol Biochem.* 21:151-60, 2008.
[37] Haase-Flielitz A et al. *JASN* 20:1393-403, 2009
[38] D.O'Sullivan and V.E.Torres in *Comprehensive Clinical Nephrology*, p.505, Feehally Floege and Johnson, Philadelphia 2007.
[39] D.M.Alscher and U.Kuhlmann in *Nephrologie*, p.521, Kuhlmann, Walb, Böhler and Luft, Stuttgart / New York 2008.

In: Nephrology – Dialysis - Transplantation
Editors: Endre Kruger and Kelemen Hahn
ISBN 978-1-60741-736-1
© 2009 Nova Science Publishers, Inc.

Chapter VIII

Plasma Exchanges Prescription for Nephrologists

Seck Sidy Mohamed and Diouf Boucar
Nephrology Department, Teaching hospital Aristide Le Dantec

Abstract

Therapeutic plasma exchanges (TPE) have been firstly performed with centrifugation devices used in blood banking procedures. Nowadays TPE are increasingly performed in intensive nephrology care units using hemodialysis generators and membrane plasma separation that ensures better efficiency and simplicity. However, prescription in different medical pathologies often depends on weak evidence-based recommendations and is guided by clinician's own experience. In this review, after recalling rationale of plasmapheresis prescription, we will discuss evidence level of most common indications of TPE in nephrology. Currently, strongest evidence-based data have found that benefit of TPE is demonstrated in diseases like haemolytic uremic syndrome, anti-glomerular basement membrane nephropathy and humoral renal allograft rejection. But this benefit is still controversed in ANCA-associated vasculitis and clearly absent in lupus nephritis. More randomized clinical trials are needed.

I. Introduction

Therapeutic plasma exchange or plasmapheresis is an extra-corporeal blood purification technique that permits to remove high molecular weight plasmatic proteins from a blood volume passing through a membrane plasma separation (MPS) or plasmafilter [1, 2]. Toxic substances thus removed from plasma might be pathogenic auto-antibodies, immune complexes, cryoglobulins, light chains from monoclonal lymphocyte proliferation, endotoxins, or cholesterol associated with lipoproteins. Plasmapheresis is expected to eliminate markedly these circulating substances from plasma in order to slow disease progression. One more benefit of plasma exchanges is activation of reticulo-endothelial system leading to better clearance of endogen proteins [3], improvement of cytotoxic treatment by stimulation of some lymphocytes clones [4], and possibility to substitute important volume of patient's plasma without overload risk. TPE are usually supportive treatment associated with immunosuppressant drugs that inhibit synthesis of new immunoglobulins. One particular case is thrombotic thrombocytopenic purpura where plasma exchange represents the cornerstone of its therapy and removes acquired auto-antibodies and the very high molecular weight von Willebrand factor (VWF).

The following paragraphs will rapidly go through soe basic notions that must be understood before prescribing TPE and review current indications in nephrology field.

II. Prescription of TPE in Nephrology: Technical Patterns

Plasma exchanges have been firstly performed with centrifugation devices used in blood banking procedures. But, utilisation of a filter that is compatible with standard hemodialysis equipment represents an increasingly popular and more efficient method of plasma separation [1, 2]. Using hemodialysis generators which are equipped with a double roller pump also permits to limit blood flow and to regulate the infusion of replacement fluid (such as albumin or fresh frozen plasma), matching its rate of return to the volume of plasma removed, thereby eliminating the risk of hypotension or fluid overload. Many aspects might be considered when prescribing plasmapheresis in a patient.

II.1. Membrane Plasma Separation (MPS)

The plasmafilter is a highly adsorbant and permeable membrane. These interesting characteristics are also responsible of one major limit: formation of "protein cake" (proteins layering on the inner surface of the membrane). During plasmapheresis, this phenomenon will rapidly limit the maximum achievable filtration rate [1]. As a result, inappropriately high transmembrane pressures will not yield higher filtration rates but will increase the tendency for the filter to clog. MPS should be operated with a limited transmembrane pressure (<75 mm Hg) and blood flow (below 150 ml/min) in order to minimize hemolysis and filter clotting [5]. The highest filtration rate is achieved at a relatively low TMP pressure of about 40 mmHg.

II.2. Vascular Access

Success of TPE depends largely on quality of vascular access. Any vascular access compatible with hemodialysis can be used since the blood flow requirements are modest. Venous access may be either two large, durable peripheral veins or a central line using a catheter with a dual lumen and is rigid enough to withstand significant flow and pressures. Typically, the blood flow rate is frequently between 100 and 150 ml/min.

II.3. Replacement Fluids

To prevent marked volume depletion during plasma exchange, different replacement fluids can be used and each has its own advantages and limits (see table I).

Table I. Different replacement fluids and their advantages

Fluids	Advantages	Disadvantages
Albumin alone	No risk of viral transmission Low risk of anaphylactoid reactions	Depletion coagulopathy Net loss of immunoglobulins High cost
Albumin and saline	The same as albumin with lower cost	The same as albumin Requirement to mix fluids in appropriate proportions (60 to 80% colloid and 20 to 40% saline)
Fresh frozen plasma	No depletion of coagulation factors or immunoglobulins	Citrate-induced hypocalcemia (paresthesias, muscle cramps) Allergic reactions (from pruritus, urticaria to severe anaphylaxis)

Fresh frozen plasma or cryosupernatant (also called cryoprecipitate-reduced or cryo-poor plasma) are more adapted in thrombotic thrombocytopenic purpura [6].

II.4. Volume of Plasma Exchange

For an adult, the following formula helps to estimate the theorical plasma volume [7]:

Estimated plasma volume (in liters) = 0.07 x weight (kg) x (1 - hematocrit)

Generally, it is enough to exchange 1 to 1.5 plasma volume per procedure. Performing more than one plasma volume exchange will increase procedure time, challenges patient tolerance, and increases the cost.

II.5. Frequency of Procedures

It is admitted that five plasma exchanges within a 7 to 10 days period remove 90% of immunoglobulins previously present in the body [8]. Additional treatments may be required if new antibody production occurs. The generally recommended frequency is one exchange every two or three days for a total of three to five procedures. Exceptions are thrombotic thrombocytopenic purpura and Goodpasture's syndrome where TPE are initially performed on a daily basis.

II.6. Anticoagulation

Many centres use heparin for anticoagulation during plasmapheresis. The recommended dosage is 5000 U [2] or 40 to 60 U/Kg [9] at the first hour followed by 1000 U/h during next hours. This dosage should be increased in patients with low hematocrit [10]. However, citrate can also be used [11] with a higher risk of side-effects due to induced hypocalcemia (see next paragraph).

II.7. Complications of Plasma Exchange Procedure

Like any extra-corporeal blood purification technique, TPE expose to many complications. These are substantially more frequent with fresh frozen plasma (FFP) than with albumin (20% versus 1.4%) [3]. Most frequent complications are citrate-induced paresthesias (due to binding of free calcium to citrate), muscle cramps, and urticaria but more serious complications, such as severe anaphylactoid reactions, can occur with administration of FFP and other plasma-containing replacement fluid [12]. The main complications are regrouped in the following table II.

Table II. Complications of plasma exchange procedure

Complications	Mechanism	Management
Hypotension	Volume depletion	Infuse additional intravascular fluid or increasing the return rate
Paresthesias	Citrate-induced hypocalcemia	Slow the rate of exchange (pump) Prophylaxis: infuse slowly one 10 ml ampul of 10% calcium chloride, 15 minutes after the start of plasma exchange
Coagulation abnormalities	Decrease in clotting factors when albumin issued as replacement fluid	Use of fresh frozen plasma in patients at high risk of bleeding
Opportunistic infections	Removal of immunoglobulins and complement	Infuse IV immunoglobulins to restore immunity
Viral transmission (HIV, Hepatitis, HTLV,etc)	Exposure to blood products (fresh frozen plasma)	Prevention by testing all products before use, hepatitis B vaccination Give large-volume plasma units collected from a single donor rather than multiple single units
Hypokaliemia in the postpheresis period	Dilution induced by albumin-based replacement fluids	Prophylaxis: add 4 mEq of potassium to each litre of albumin
Anaphylactic reactions	Use of fresh frozen plasma	Stop procedure Resuscitation measures
Drug removal	Removal of highly protein-bounded drugs	Administer the drug after a plasma exchange

Other complications such as problems with vascular catheters, pulmonary embolism, metabolic alkalosis or flushing due to angiotensin converting enzyme inhibitors can occur during plasma exchange procedure and threaten patient's life.

The whole mortality rate of plasmapheresis is around 0.05 % [13]. Respiratory and cardiovascular complications are the most common causes of death [14].

Anaphylaxis, vascular complications, hepatitis, sepsis, and thrombosis are other less reported causes of death.

III. Current Indications of Plasma Exchanges in Nephrology

There is currently any evidence-based international guideline for prescription of TPE in medicine. Thus, main indications are variable from one country to another. Chronic inflammatory neuropathies, myasthenia gravis and thrombocytopenic thrombotic purpura are the most recognized indications in USA and Canada [3, 15].

Despite these variations, indications of TPE might be rational in diseases that fit at least one of the following conditions:

- The substance to be removed should be sufficiently large (molecular weight greater than 15,000) so that it cannot be easily removed by less expensive purification techniques such as hemofiltration or high-flux hemodialysis.
- The substance to be removed must have a sufficiently long half-life, so that extracorporeal removal is much more rapid than endogenous clearance pathways.
- The substance to be removed must be acutely toxic and resistant to conventional therapy, so that the rapid elimination from the extracellular fluid by TPE is indicated.

Given the complexity and expense of the procedure, guidelines are needed to provide a framework for clinical decisions regarding the use of TPE [16].

The following paragraphs will discuss the most common indication of TPE in nephrology field.

III.1. Thrombotic Thrombocytopenic Purpura-Hemolytic Uremic Syndrome (TTP-HUS)

II.3.1. In adults

In HUS plasma exchanges can reverse platelets consumption and then inhibits development of thrombus that are responsible of organ damages [17, 18].

Moreover, in particular etiologies of atypical HUS, plasmapheresis is used in conjunction with plasma infusion that helps substituting a missing enzyme, and immunosuppressive drugs (eg, steroids, rituximab) which reduce the production of auto-antibodies.

In clinical medicine, results from randomized controlled trials found no additional therapy proven to increase efficacy over plasma exchange for patients with TTP [19]. Studies have also suggested a more effectiveness of TPE with fresh frozen plasma versus plasma infusion alone that expose volume overload. Plasmapheresis induces a better remission and survival rates at six months compared to plasma infusion, and higher mortality rate is reported in non-responders patients [16, 20]. Despite results from one retrospective study in which high doses of plasma infusions (25 to 30 mL/kg per day) were temporarily effective in some patients [21], they might be restricted to emergency treatment of patients when plasmapheresis is not immediately accessible.

Plasma exchange may be initiated even if the diagnosis of TTP-HUS is not yet confirmed [22]. If an alternative diagnosis is subsequently discovered then TPE should be stopped. Recommended schedule is one daily exchange until normalization of platelet count and serum lactate dehydrogenase (LDH) concentration [22, 23]. It is also recommended to exchange one estimated plasma volume during each procedure [24]. Generally, one to two weeks are required to induce remission, but the variability between patients is large and unpredictable [25].

Recovery of renal function is unpredictable and often incomplete. Duration of TPE maintenance once thrombocytopenia and hemolysis have been corrected is unknown. After end of plasmapheresis relapses are frequent particularly in atypical HUS secondary to abnomalities in complement pathway regulatory proteins or deficiency in von Willebrand factor metalloprotease (ADAMTS 13) where plasma infusions have an important role [26]. Post-infectious HUS is rare in adults and there are no evidence on benefit of plasmapheresis in this indication.

II.3.2. In children

There are not enough studies assessing TPE in post-infectious HUS and results are not clear [27, 28]. In children with associated neurologic symptoms (TTP-HUS), TPE may be useful by analogy with TTP in adults. Meta-analysis reported that plasmapheresis is the most effective intervention for TTP and plasma manipulation offers no additional benefit over simple supportive therapy in HUS [19] but this conclusion should be carefuly taken because trials considered in this meta-analysis did not make difference between causes of of TTP-HUS [28].

In absence of relevant studies management of atypical HUS in children is currently extrapolated from adults. Plasma infusion have demonstrated good outcomes in atypical HUS due to complement factor deficiency [29].

III.2. Renal vasculitis

III.2.1. Anti-Glomerular Basement Membrane Disease

One of the most widely used indication of TPE is Goodpasture' syndrome where it represents an essential part of the treatment in association with corticosteroids and immunosuppressants. Plasmapheresis decreases rapidly serum level circulating anti-GBM antibodies and reduces serum creatinine by half [30]. For patients with severe renal damage (serum creatinine ≥ 600 μmol/l), plasmapheresis does not improve renal function but it is the best therapy in presence of alveolar haemorrhage. Authors recommend daily TPE with albumin 4% (60 ml/kg weight) as substitution fluid and during 14 days at least [31].

III.2.2. Pauci-Immune Renal Vasculitis

Many randomized clinical trials have assessed benefits of TPE in patients with pauci-immune glomerulonephritis. Prospective studies have not demonstrated any advantage of adding plasma exchanges to immunosuppressive drugs alone [16, 32]. At the other hand, one recent study from European Vasculitis Study Group (EUVAS) showed that TPE improved renal function in patients with severe renal damage requiring dialysis [33]. In their study, 137 patients with a diagnosis of ANCA-associated vasculitis confirmed by renal biopsy and serum creatinine >500 μmol/l (5.8 mg/dl) were randomly assigned to receive seven plasma exchanges (n = 70) or 3000 mg of intravenous methylprednisolone (n = 67). Both groups received oral cyclophosphamide and oral prednisolone. Plasmapheresis group showed better rate of renal recovery and lower risk of ESRD. However, patient survival and severe adverse events were similar. In patients with less severe renal dysfunction prescription of TPE should be discussed carefully because there are no data supporting their superiority to standard therapy [34]. In other necrotizing vasculitis such as Churg-Strauss syndrome, microscopic polyangitis and renal-limited vasculitis there is not enough evidence to recommend TPE use but patients with severe acute renal failure may take profit from this therapy [35].

III.2.3.Other Renal Vasculitis

III.2.3.1. Systemic Lupus Erythematosus

Many prospective studies have assessed TPE in treatment of patients with systemic lupus [34, 36]. None of them have demonstrated benefit of plasmapheresis for management of lupus nephropathy. In a randomized trial including patients with severe lupus nephritis, Lewis and coll. compared plasmapheresis versus corticosteroids and cyclophosphamide but they did not find any difference on renal function and disease prognosis between two groups [37]. The Lupus Plasmapheresis Study Group (LPSG) demonstrated that adding plasmapheresis to IV cyclophosphamide bolus was not better than cyclophosphamide alone [38, 39]. Current indications of plasmapheresis in systemic lupus are:

- Resistance to usual therapy including corticosteroids and immunosuppressive drugs (rescue treatment).
- Neurolupus: even without anticardiolipin antibody, TPE might improve neurologic functions in patients with neurolupus associating coma or motor impairment.
- Catastrophic antiphospholipid antibody syndrome in combination with anticoagulation.
- Renal injury during associated thrombotic microangiopathy.

III.2.3.2. Periarteritis Nodosa (PAN)

In HBV-associated periarteritis nodosa, TPE are combined with antiviral drugs as first line therapy. This protocol ensures remission for majority of patients within two or three months and blockage of viral replication for more than half of cases [31].

III.2.3.3. Mixed Cryoglobulinemia

Plasmapheresis is also suggested in combination with interferon alpha in vasculitis involving severe renal impairment and/or other life threatening organ damages (central nervous system, airways and digestive, severe mononeuropathy) [4]. Therapy is often initiated at three or more litres, using prewarmed tubing, bags and other reagents to avoid cryoprecipitation in the instruments, and exchanges are performed three times per week for three weeks or until the resolution of a life-threatening state. Recent data suggest prescribing three TPE per week during first three weeks, followed by two exchanges per week, and finally one exchange every week or couple of weeks according to therapeutic response [23]. However results are often not so good. Eradication of HCV occurs in a few patients, and relapses are frequent.

III.3. Paraproteinemia

Studies assessing TPE in patients with acute renal failure due to myeloma are conflicting and some patients clearly improve without plasmapheresis [40, 41]. However, substantial benefit in renal outcomes has been shown in some studies that enrolled patients with circulating free light chains in the plasma or significant Bence Jones proteinuria. According to most recent studies, plasmapheresis represents an important adjunct therapy in management of patients with suspected myeloma cast nephropathy in conjunction with chemotherapy [40, 42]. By decreasing markedly toxic free light chains from the plasma, TPE improves rate of renal function recovery and dialysis independence [43]. Small-sized studies did not find any benefit of TPE in patients with acute renal failure at the onset of myeloma but diagnosis of cast nephropathy was not biopsy proven and a composite outcome of death, dialysis dependence, or glomerular filtration rate was used [41, 44]. One ongoing trial includes patients with severe cast nephropathyis evaluating efficacy of hemodialysis with high cut-off polyamide membrane on renal outcome [45].

In practice, whenever cast nephropathy is strongly suspected, plasmapheresis may be initiated on the basis of high levels of free monoclonal light chains in the serum or urine, even in the absence of a renal biopsy. Partial replacement with fresh frozen plasma rather than albumin can prevent bleeding if renal biopsy has recently been performed or prior to central catheter removal. The usual frequency of exchanges is five to seven exchanges within seven to ten days. However, duration of TPE should be guided by serum free light chain levels. Recurrent light chain accumulation should be monitored typically one to two days after completing the initial course of plasma exchange. In case of recurrent light chain production TPE can be continued for one more course.

TPE are also indicated in hyperviscosity syndrome associated with other dysproteinemias [42].

III.4. Renal Transplantation

In renal transplantation, indications of plasmapheresis have evolved these last decades. Plasma exchanges are used in management of antibody-mediated rejection (AMR), desensitization protocols in highly immunized patients and recurrence of glomerular diseases on renal allograft.

- Management of antibody-mediated rejection:

AMR is a real challenge in renal transplantation because it can lead to rapid allograft dysfunction. It is generally less responsive to conventional anti-rejection therapy and results in poor allograft survival [46]. Adding plasma exchanges to IV immunoglobulin is an interesting and promising therapeutic strategy in sensitized patients with strong donor-specific antibodies but efficacy of such protocols has to be confirmed in more randomized clinical trials [47].

Although, TPE can lower rapidly circulating donor specific antigens in patients with acute AMR [48], they do not prevent onset of chronic AMR and shortened graft survival [49]. Also, required number of plasma exchanges is not clearly defined (from 2 to 15 according to available data [15]). It seems that a short interval between transplantation and the acute rejection onset correlates more with good response to plasmapheresis than number of exchanges [50].

- Prevention of antibody-mediated rejection in graft recipients at risk of antibody (highly HLA sensitized patients or recipient of ABO mismatch graft) [47]:

Typically TPE are performed before transplantation in desensitization protocol in many countries [51, 52]. They are associated with anti-CD20 antibodies or IV immunoglobulins for better removal of antibodies in highly HLA-sensitized patients [52]. In highly HLA sensitized patients, TPE permit to have more negative cross-match than IV Ig but they do not eliminate risk of AMR [53]. Widely used protocols are based on combination of TPE and IV Ig that have proven reduction of AMR by 7% in high risk patients [54].

- Recurrence of certain nephropathies after renal transplantation:

Plamapheresis are essentially indicated in relapse of idiopathic focal glomerulosclerosis (FSGS) on renal allograft, HUS and less frequently particular types of membranous glomerulopathy [55, 56]

In early recurrence of FSGS, TPE should be continued until stabilisation of proteinuria below 1g/24h [57]. In late recurrence of diseases, TPE are used in combination with immunosuppressive drugs [58, 59]

Conclusion

Plasma exchange therapy is increasingly used in different situations in nephrology. By reducing markedly immunoglobulins, it represents a powerful therapeutic option in management of patients with severe acute renal failure due to vasculitis, cast nephropathy and antibody mediated rejection after renal transplantation. Utilisation of dialysis devices has simplified the procedure that becomes more accessible to nephrologists in intensive renal care units. However, plasmapheresis remains a burdensome and costly therapy and indications might be discussed in each case according to potential proven benefits and complications. Except in hemolytic uremic syndrome, plasma exchange therapy is never systematic and must be combined with corticosteroids and/or immunosuppressant drugs. Randomized controlled trials are needed to precise their place in renal care.

References

[1] Gurland HJ, Lysaght MJ, Samtleben W, Schmidt B. Comparative evaluation of filters used in membrane plasmapheresis. *Nephron.* 1984; 36(3):173-82.

[2] Gerhardt RE, Ntoso KA, Koethe JD, Lodge S, Wolf CJ. Acute plasma separation with hemodialysis equipment. *J. Am. Soc. Nephrol.* 1992; 2(9):1455-8.

[3] Lockwood CM, Worlledge S, Nicholas A, Cotton C, Peters DK. Reversal of impaired splenic function in patients with nephritis or vasculitis (or both) by plasma exchange. *N. Engl. J. Med.* 1979; 300(10):524-30.

[4] Schroeder JO, Euler HH, Loffler H. Synchronization of plasmapheresis and pulse cyclophosphamide in severe systemic lupus erythematosus. *Ann. Intern. Med.* 1987; 107(3):344-6.

[5] Petitpas D, Ould-Zein S, Korach JM. What are the indications for plasma exchanges in autoimmune diseases ? The registry of Société Française d'Hémaphérèse. *Transfusion and Apheresis Science* 2007; 36:173-7.

[6] Rock G, Shumak KH, Sutton DM, Buskard NA, Nair RC. Cryosupernatant as replacement fluid for plasma exchange in thrombotic thrombocytopenic purpura. Members of the Canadian Apheresis Group. *Br. J. Haematol.* 1996; 94(2):383-6.

[7] Kaplan AA. A simple and accurate method for prescribing plasma exchange. *ASAIO Trans* 1990; 36(3):597-9.

[8] Keller AJ, Urbaniak SJ. Intensive plasma exchange on the cell separator: Effects on serum immunoglobulins and complement components. *Br. J. Haematol.* 1978; 38:531.

[9] Price CA. Therapeutic plasma exchange in a dialysis unit. *ANNA J* 1987; 14:103.

[10] Frasca GM, Buscaroli A, Borgnino LC, Vangelista A. Optimization of heparin anticoagulation during membrane plasma separation. *Int. J. Artif. Organs* 1988; 11(4):313-6.

[11] Ilamathi E, Kirsch M, Moore B, Finger M. Citrate anticoagulation during plasmapheresis using standard hemodialysis equipment. *Semin. Dial.* 1993; 6:268.

[12] Sutton DM, Nair RC, Rock G. Complications of plasma exchange. *Transfusion* 1989; 29(2):124-7.

[13] Mokrzycki MH; Kaplan AA. Therapeutic plasma exchange: complications and management. *Am. J. Kidney Dis.* 1994; 23(6):817-27.

[14] Walker RH. Technical Manual (11th Ed), American Association of Blood Banks, Bethesda 1993. p.37.

[15] Clark WF, Rock GA, Buskard N, Shumak K, LeBlond P, Anderson D, Sutton DM. Therapeutic plasma exchange: an update from the Canadian Apheresis Group. *Ann. Intern. Med.* 1999; 131(6):453-62.

[16] von Baeyer H. Plasmapheresis in immune hematology: review of clinical outcome data with respect to evidence-based medicine and clinical experience. *Therap. Apher. Dial* 2003; 7(1):127-40.

[17] Moake JL. Thrombotic microangiopathies. N Engl J Med 2002; 347(8):589-600.

[18] Kaplan AA. Therapeutic apheresis for cancer related hemolytic uremic syndrome. *Ther Apher* 2000; 4(3):201-6.

[19] Michael M, Elliott EJ, Craig JC, Ridley G, Hodson EM. Interventions for hemolytic uremic syndrome and thrombotic thrombocytopenic purpura: A Systematic Review of Randomized Controlled Trials. *Am. J. Kidney Dis* 2009; 53(2):259-72.

[20] Rock GA, Shumak KH, Buskard NA, Blanchette VS, Kelton JG, Nair RC, Spasoff RA. Comparison of plasma exchange with plasma infusion in the treatment of thrombotic thrombocytopenic purpura. Canadian Apheresis Study Group. *N. Engl. J. Med.* 1991; 325(6):393-7.

[21] Coppo P, Bussel A, Charrier S, Adrie C, Galicier L, et al. High-dose plasma infusion versus plasma exchange as early treatment of thrombotic thrombocytopenic purpura/hemolytic-uremic syndrome. *Medicine (Baltimore)* 2003; 82(1):27-38.

[22] George JN. How I treat patients with thrombotic thrombocytopenic purpura-hemolytic uremic syndrome. *Blood* 2000; 96(4):1223-9.

[23] Cacoub P, Sène D, Saadoun D. Cryoglobulinemia. *Rev. Méd. Interne* 2008; 29:200-8.

[24] George JN, Gilcher RO, Smith JW, Chandler L, Duvall D, Ellis C. Thrombotic thrombocytopenic purpura-hemolytic uremic syndrome: diagnosis and management. *J. Clin. Apheresis* 1998; 13(3):120-5.

[25] Ruggenenti P, Noris M, Remuzzi G. Thrombotic microangiopathy, hemolytic uremic syndrome, and thrombotic thrombocytopenic purpura. *Kidney Int.* 2001; 60(3):831-46.

[26] Noris M, Remuzzi G. Thrombotic microangiopathy: What not to learn from a meta-analysis. *Nature Reviews Nephrology* 2009; 5 :186-188.

[27] Slavicek J, Puretic Z, Novak M, Sarnavka V, Beniak V, Glavas-Boras S, Thune S. The role of plasma exchange in the treatment of severe forms of haemolytic-uremic syndrome in childhood. *Artif. Organs* 1995; 19(6):506-10.

[28] Boyce TG, Swerdlow DL, Griffin PM. Escherichia coli O157:H7 and the haemolytic-uremic syndrome. *N. Engl. J. Med.* 1995; 333(6):364-8.

[29] Davin JC, Strain L, Goodship T H. Plasma therapy in atypical haemolytic uremic syndrome: lessons from a family with a factor H mutation. *Pediatr. Nephrol.* 2008; 23:1517-21.

[30] Johnson J, Moore J, Austin H, Balow J, Antonovych T, Wilson C. Therapy of anti-glomerular basement membrane antibody disease. Analysis of prognostic significance of clinical, pathologic, and treatment factors. *Medicine (Baltimore)* 1985; 64:219-27.

[31] Guillevin L. Plasma exchange: their current place in the treatment of systemic diseases. *Réanimation* 2002; 11:359-65.

[32] Glöckner WM, Sieberth HG, Wichmann HE. Plasma exchange and immunosuppression in rapidly progressive glomerulonephritis: a controlled, multi-center study. *Clin. Nephrol.* 1988; 29:1-8.

[33] Jayne DRW, Gaskin G, Rasmussen N, Abramowicz D, Ferrario F, Guillevin L et al. Randomized Trial of Plasma Exchange or High-Dosage Methylprednisolone as Adjunctive Therapy for Severe Renal Vasculitis. *J. Am. Soc. Nephrol.* 2007; 18:2180-8.

[34] David J Salant. Intravenous methylprednisolone or plasma exchange for adjunctive therapy of severe renal vasculitis? Nat. Clin. Pract. Nephrol. 2008; 4:14-15.

[35] Walters G, Willis NS, Craig JC. Interventions for renal vasculitis in adults. *Cochrane Database of Systematic Reviews* 2008, Issue 3. Art. No.: CD003232. DOI: 10.1002/14651858.CD003232.pub2.

[36] French Cooperative group. A randomized trial of plasma exchange in severe acute systemic lupus erythematosus. *Plasma Ther Transfus Technol* 1985; 6:535-9.

[37] Wei N, Klippel JH, Huston DP, Hall RP, Lawley TC, Balow JE, et al. Randomized trial of plasma exchange in mild systemic lupus erythematosus. *Lancet* 1983; 1:17-22.

[38] Lewis EJ. A controlled trial of plasmapheresis in severe lupus nephritis. *N. Engl. J. Med.* 1992; 326:1373-9.

[39] Euler HH, Schroeder JO. Antibody depletion and cytotoxic drug therapy in severe systemic lupus erythematosus. *Transfus Sci.* 1992; 13:167-84.

[40] Durie BG, Kyle RA, Belch A, Bensinger W, Blade J, Boccadoro M, et al. Myeloma management guidelines: a consensus report from the Scientific Advisors of the International Myeloma Foundation. *Hematol J.* 2003; 4(6):379-98.

[41] Cserti C, Haspel R, Stowell C, Dzik W. Light-chain removal by plasmapheresis in myeloma-associated renal failure. *Transfusion* 2007; 47(3):511-4.

[42] Kaplan AA. Therapeutic apheresis for the renal complications of multiple myeloma and the dysglobulinemias. *Ther. Apher* 2001; 5(3):171-5.

[43] Leung N, Gertz MA, Zeldenrust SR, Rajkumar SV, Dispenzieri A, et al. Improvement of cast nephropathy with plasma exchange depends on the diagnosis and on reduction of serum free light chains. *Kidney Int* 2008; 73(11):1282-8.

[44] Clark WF, Stewart AK, Rock GA, Sternbach M, Sutton DM, Barrett BJ, Heidenheim AP, Garg AX, Churchill DN. Plasma exchange when myeloma presents as acute renal failure: a randomized, controlled trial. *Ann. Intern. Med.* 2005; 143(11):777-84.

[45] Hutchison CA, Cook M, Heyne N, Weisel K, Billingham L, Bradwell A, Cockwell P. European trial of free light chain removal by extended haemodialysis in cast nephropathy (EuLITE): A randomised control trial. *Trials* 2008; 9:55.

[46] Sureshkumar KK, Hussain SM, Carpenter BJ, Sandroni SE, Marcus RJ. Antibody-mediated rejection following renal transplantation. *Expert Opin. Pharmacother* 2007; 8(7):913-21.

[47] Akalin E, Dinavahi R, Friedlander R, Ames S, de Boccardo G, Sehgal V, Schröppel B, et al. Addition of plasmapheresis decreases the incidence of acute antibody-mediated rejection in sensitized patients with strong donor-specific antibodies. *Clin. J. Am. Soc. Nephrol.* 2008; 3(4):1160-7.

[48] Rocha PN, Butterly DW, Greenberg A, Reddan DN, Tuttle-Newhall D, Collins BH, et al. Benefical effects of plasmapheresis and intravenous immunoglobulin on allograft survival of patients with acute humoral rejection. *Transplantation* 2003; 75:1490-5.

[49] Gloor J, Cosio F, Lager DJ, Stegall MD. The spectrum of antibody-mediated renal allograft injury: implications for treatment. *Am. J. Transplant* 2008; 8(7):1367-73.

[50] Al-Badr W, Kallogjeri D, Madaraty K, Oliver D, Bastani B, Grossman BJ. Retrospective review of the outcome of plasma exchange and aggressive medical therapy in antibody mediated rejection of renal allografts: A single centre experience. *J. Clin. Apher.* 2008; 23(6):178-82.

[51] Ichimaru N, Takahara S. Japan's experience with living-donor kidney transplantation across ABO barriers. *Nat. Clin. Pract. Nephrol.* 2008; 4(12):682-92.

[52] Jordan SC, Peng A, Vo AA. Therapeutic strategies in management of the highly HLA-sensitized and ABO-incompatible Transplant Recipients. *Contrib. Nephrol.* 2009; 162:13-26.

[53] Stegall MD, Gloor J, Winters JL, Moore SB, Degoey S. A comparison of plasmapheresis versus high-dose IVIG desensitization in renal allograft recipients with high levels of donor specific alloantibody. *Am. J. Transplant* 2006; 6(2):346-51.

[54] Dragun D, Rudolph B. Novelties in diagnostics and therapy of antibody mediated rejection. *Nephrol. Dial Transplant* 2007; 22 (8):50-3.

[55] Couser W. Recurrent glomerulonephritis in the renal allograft: an update of selected areas. *Exp. Clin. Transplant* 2005; 3(1):283-8.

[56] Choy BY, Chan TM, Lai KN. Recurrent glomerulonephritis after kidney transplantation. *Am. J. Transplant* 2006; 6(11):2535-42.

[57] Deegens JK, Andresdottir MB, Croockewit S, Wetzels JF. Plasma exchange improves graft survival in patients with recurrent focal glomerulosclerosis after renal transplant. *Transplant Int.* 2004; 17(3):151-7.

[58] Cheong HI, Han HW, Park HW, Ha IS, Han KS, Lee HS, Kim SJ, Choi Y. Early recurrent nephrotic syndrome after renal transplantation in children with focal segmental glomerulosclerosis. *Nephrol. Dial Transplant* 2000; 15(1):78-81.

[59] Hariharan S. Recurrent and de novo diseases after renal transplantation. *Semin. Dial* 2000; 13(3):195-9.

In: Nephrology – Dialysis - Transplantation
Editors: Endre Kruger and Kelemen Hahn

ISBN 978-1-60741-736-1
© 2009 Nova Science Publishers, Inc.

Chapter IX

The Role of Macrophages in Obstructive Nephropathy

Masashi Nishida* and Kenji Hamaoka
Department of Pediatric Cardiology and Nephrology,
Kyoto Prefectural University of Medicine
Graduate School of Medical Science, Kyoto (Japan)

Abstract

Macrophages have classically been recognized as active players that mediate and promote renal fibrosis. However, several recent studies including ours have suggested a beneficial anti-fibrotic role of infiltrating macrophages in some settings of obstructive nephropathy. Furthermore, recent investigations indicating that macrophages can be functionally distinguished into two broad phenotypes, and that macrophages play a role in both inflammation and repair during the process of inflammatory responses, has superseded the classical injurious view of macrophages. As a result, the exact role of interstitial macrophages upon various facets of renal fibrosis has emerged as an important challenge that needs to be addressed. In this article, we focus upon the potentially anti-fibrotic actions of infiltrating macrophages in obstructive nephropathy and discuss the potential mechanisms that may regulate the effect of macrophages upon renal interstitial fibrosis.

Introduction

Obstructive nephropathy describes renal disease that leads to hydronephrosis caused by urinary tract obstruction. Although obstructive nephropathy is a common pathology in infants

* Corresponding author: Masashi Nishida, M.D., Ph.D. Department of Pediatric Cardiology and Nephrology, Kyoto Prefectural University of Medicine Graduate School of Medical Science, Kawaramachi-Hirokoji, Kamigyoku, Kyoto 602-8566, Japan. Phone: +81 75 251 5832; Fax: +81 75 251 5833. E-mail: mnishida@koto.kpu-m.ac.jp

with congenital urinary tract abnormalities, and the primary cause of end-stage renal disease in children, an increasingly used and popular animal model of obstructive nephropathy is complete unilateral ureteral obstruction (UUO). UUO is a well-established model of nonimmunological progressive renal interstitial fibrosis, and results in many pathophysiological events related to renal interstitial fibrosis within 1 week following ureteral ligation that encompass many aspects of other kidney disease models [1].

Chronic inflammation in the renal tubulointerstitial compartment with subsequent progressive interstitial fibrosis is characterized by inflammatory cell infiltrates in the early stage. Cells of monocyte/macrophage lineage are always present and often predominate cell type among infiltrating cells both in experimental models and human renal diseases, and the presence of macrophages correlates with the degree of renal fibrosis. Thus, these infiltrating macrophages have been considered to be an active player that promote fibrosis [2]. Also in the UUO model, interstitial macrophage infiltration is evident soon after ureteral ligation [3] and these macrophages have been recognized as playing a central role in the inflammatory response and subsequent progression of interstitial fibrosis. However, several recent studies have suggested a beneficial anti-fibrotic role of infiltrating macrophages in some settings of obstructive nephropathy [4-9]. Furthermore, recent investigations have highlighted new roles for macrophages in the biology of inflammation and fibrosis and extended the role of macrophages in both inflammation and tissue repair [10-15]. In this article, we discuss on the possible regulatory role of infiltrating macrophages in renal injury and repair during renal fibrosis induced by UUO.

The Different Stages in the Development of Obstructive Nephropathy

The pathological changes in the kidney following UUO include cellular infiltration that consists mostly with macrophages, tubular proliferation and apoptosis, epithelial-mesenchymal transdifferentiation (EMT), myofibroblast accumulation, increased extracellular matrix (ECM) deposition, and tubular atrophy [1]. These pathological changes represent the different stages in the development of obstructive nephropathy in the time frame after UUO. An increase in the number of interstitial macrophages is evident as early as 4 hours after ureteral ligation. Interstitial macrophage number increases rapidly in the first 24 hours prior to the development of fibrosis, and plateaus at a level approximately 10-fold higher than normal levels until day 3 [3]. Although macrophages constitute the predominant infiltrating cell population in acutely obstructed kidneys, increased numbers of T lymphocytes are also evident after 24 hours of obstruction though neither B lymphocytes nor neutrophils are observed. Interstitial macrophage numbers further increase at 96 hours after ureteral ligation following the emergence of established fibrosis. Thus, the degree of macrophage infiltration at 14 days is much greater than that at 5 days after obstruction [4]. This biphasic pattern in the increase of interstitial macrophages, i.e., an initial rapid increase during the first 24 hours after UUO and the second phase following 72 hours after UUO suggests that discussion of the role of interstitial macrophages in obstructive nephropathy should take into account the time frame after UUO.

Recent studies have demonstrated multiple molecules that direct circulating monocytes to the site of disease. These include selectin-mediated rolling, and integrin-mediated adhesion of monocytes on the surface of endothelial cells, followed by transendothelial and subendothelial migration of these monocytes. Various kinds of chemokines that direct monocytes to the site of disease have also been demonstrated on cells such as tubular epithelial cells and in peritubular capillaries. These include monocyte chemoattractant protein-1 (MCP-1) and regulated upon activation, normal T cell expressed and secreted (RANTES). Targeted deletion of these individual molecules or their counter-receptors primarily interrupted the initial phase of macrophage infiltration following UUO and resulted in reduced renal fibrosis [16]. Systemic depletion of macrophages by the administration of liposome-encapsulated clodronate interrupted the initial interstitial macrophage infiltration and resulted in a decreased renal fibrosis in a rat UUO model [17]. Thus, the results of these studies suggest that the initial phase of macrophage infiltration may promote renal fibrosis.

Functional Heterogeneity of Macrophages in Obstructive Nephropathy

The contribution of macrophages to the pathogenesis of renal fibrosis has been widely recognized, and indeed, interrupting the initial phase of macrophage infiltration following UUO results in decreased interstitial fibrosis. However, macrophages are originally a heterogeneous population of cells that belongs to the mononuclear phagocyte system, and there is compelling evidence that they also participate in the resolution of injury and promote tissue repair. In this context, several previous studies have also indicated an inverse correlation between the number of interstitial macrophages and the degree of fibrosis in obstructive nephropathy thereby suggesting a potential renoprotective role of macrophages in renal fibrosis. We previously reported the inverse correlation between interstitial macrophage number and interstitial fibrosis in mice that had received a bone marrow transplant from angiotensin II type 1 receptor null (*Agtr1 -/-*) mice [4]. In this model, it has been suggested that suppressed macrophage infiltration and accelerated renal fibrosis are associated with impaired macrophage functions such as migrating activity and phagocytic activity of *Agtr1 -/-* macrophages. We found a similar relationship in mice that either underwent cyclophosphamide-mediated peripheral macrophage depletion [7] or were treated with matrix metalloproteinase (MMP)-2 inhibitor [9] at day 14, but not at day 5, following UUO. In mice that had macrophage depletion by cyclophosphamide treatment, adoptive transfer of bone marrow-derived macrophages to these mice resulted in an amelioration of renal fibrosis [7]. In mice that were treated with a MMP-2 inhibitor, it has been suggested that suppressed macrophage infiltration and accelerated renal fibrosis in these mice is associated with decreased macrophage migrating activity toward the degradation products of ECM [9]. In urokinase-type plasminogen activator receptor null (*uPAR -/-*) mice, Zhang et al. demonstrated increased renal fibrosis and suppressed macrophage infiltration at day 14, but not at day 3, after UUO [5]. They suggested that the absence of scavenging receptor of *uPAR -/-* macrophages resulted in the delayed clearance of pro-fibrotic molecules. In a mouse model of reversal of ureteral obstruction (R-UUO), Cochrane et al. reported that although interstitial matrix expansion and kidney collagen concentration was markedly decreased at 6 weeks following R-UUO, interstitial macrophage infiltration still persisted at a level comparable with that of 2 weeks after R-UUO [6]. In this study, significant numbers of macrophages were associated with areas of active remodeling in the kidneys after R-UUO suggesting a role for macrophages in both renal injury and repair. Additionally, Pecly et al. reported that administration of low molecular weight heparin in the rat UUO model reduced collagen content with an increased number of infiltrating macrophages in the obstructed kidney 14 days after UUO [8]. They suggested an effect upon the activation of heparin-binding proteins expressed by circulating monocytes or the macrophage chemotactic factor midkine that is expressed by tubular epithelial cells in the diseased kidney. In all of these reports, the inverse correlation between interstitial macrophage number and the degree of fibrosis was noted at the later stage of UUO (day 14) and we should therefore consider the possible renoprotective role for macrophages that infiltrate in the later phase after UUO.

Interstitial Macrophages as Regulators of Inflammatory and Fibrotic Processes

Recent work indicates that, in response to disease status, inflammatory monocytes are recruited and undergo differentiation into two broad but distinct phenotypes of macrophages based on cell surface markers and cytokine profile that are categorized as either classically activated (M1) macrophages or alternatively activated (M2) macrophages [10-15]. Activation of M1 macrophages are induced by the Th-1 lymphokine interferon (IFN)-γ, bacterial and fungal cell wall components or degraded matrix. In contrast, activation of M2 macrophages are induced by Th-2 lymphokines such as interleukin (IL)-4, IL-10, IL-13 and transforming growth factor (TGF)-β, anti-inflammatory agents such as corticosteroids as well as the phagocytosis of apoptotic cells [18]. M1 and M2 macrophages mediate contrasting and complementary functions in tissue fibrosis. For example, M1 macrophages may induce apoptosis of host tissue cells through the release of proinflammatory mediators such as tumor necrosis factor (TNF)-α [19] and nitric oxide (NO) in rodents [20] thereby inducing tissue injury. Indeed, tubular epithelial cells represent a target of macrophage-induced apoptosis in the obstructed kidney [21]. These apoptotic cells are rapidly recognized and phagocytes by macrophages with this process promoting differentiation into M2 macrophages [19, 22]. Macrophages reprogrammed by apoptotic cell ingestion or exposure to anti-inflammatory cytokines act to dampen inflammation by the secretion of cytokines such as IL-10 and TGF-β, and appear to be highly pro-fibrogenic and contribute to tissue remodeling where increased ECM deposition predominates. Indeed, M2 macrophages produce large amounts of TGF-β [22] and can induce myofibroblast proliferation [23]. M2 macrophages also produce arginase-1, which inhibits the generation of proinflammatory NO [11], and express the IL-1 receptor antagonist, which inhibits proinflammatory cytokine IL-1 [12]. The mannose receptor, Ym1 (chitinase-like lectin), and RELM-α (resistin-like secreted protein-also known as FIZZ1 [found in inflammatory zone 1]) are also markers of M2 macrophages [24].

In contrast, M1 macrophages produce MMPs [23, 25] and can also induce myofibroblasts to produce MMPs [26] that promotes ECM degradation and facilitates the resolution of fibrosis. Furthermore, MMPs may contribute to the resolution of fibrosis by stimulating myofibroblast apoptosis [27].

Although MMPs may induce basement membrane injury and promote EMT of renal tubular cells and renal fibrosis [28], it is of interest that early inhibition of MMP-2 activity in experimental allograft nephropathy ameliorated fibrosis whereas MMP-2 inhibition in the setting of established fibrosis resulted in more severe allograft nephropathy [29]. Thus, this stimulation of the production of MMPs by M1 macrophages during the later stages of fibrosis may shift the equilibrium towards degradation and play an important anti-fibrotic role.

Although the contribution of these two phenotypes of macrophages at each stage of the fibrotic process still remains to be elucidated, Duffield et al. used a conditional monocyte/macrophage ablation system in a mouse model of liver fibrosis and clearly demonstrated the presence of two distinct macrophage phenotypes in the progression and resolution of liver fibrosis in vivo [30]. Macrophage depletion during progressive inflammatory fibrosis ameliorated scarring and reduced myofibroblast numbers whilst macrophage depletion during the recovery phase led to a failure of matrix degradation and persistent scarring.

Recent reports also indicate that macrophage-derived galectin-3 is required for TGF-β-mediated myofibroblast activation and matrix production in hepatic fibrosis [31] and obstructive nephropathy [32]. Furthermore, classical macrophage activation with IFN-γ and lipopolysaccharide (LPS) inhibits galectin-3 expression whereas galectin-3 is expressed and released by macrophages with M2 phenotypic markers with galectin-3 promoting M2 macrophage activation [33]. Thus, macrophages may regulate tissue fibrosis via galectin-3 with the production of galectin-3 being distinctively regulated by the phenotype of macrophages.

Possible Roles of Interstitial Macrophages in Obstructive Nephropathy

The proposed role of macrophages in renal fibrosis of obstructed kidneys is depicted in Figure 1. Following UUO, monocytes recruited to the interstitium differentiate into M1 (classically activated) macrophages following stimulation of Th-1-derived cytokines such as IFN-γ. M1 macrophages produce pro-inflammatory mediators (TNF-α, NO) that may induce tubular epithelial cell apoptosis and tissue injury. The differentiation to M2 (alternatively activated) macrophages may be induced by apoptotic cell phagocytosis or Th-2-derived cytokines such as IL-13 or IL-4. Apoptotic cell phagocytosis by M1 macrophages modulates their phenotype and generates macrophages with many features of M2 macrophages. M2 macrophages generate anti-inflammatory cytokines such as TGF-β and galectin-3 that result in myofibroblast activation, proliferation and ECM deposition. ECM accumulation and matrix degradation products stimulate monocyte recruitment and their differentiation into M1 macrophages, which produce MMPs that can promote ECM degradation and potentially induce apoptosis of myofibroblasts. Tubular epithelial cells may also produce TGF-β and MMPs. The ECM degradation products may induce further migration of M1 macrophages, and these matrix degradation products and apoptotic debris are possibly removed by phagocytosis of M1 macrophages.

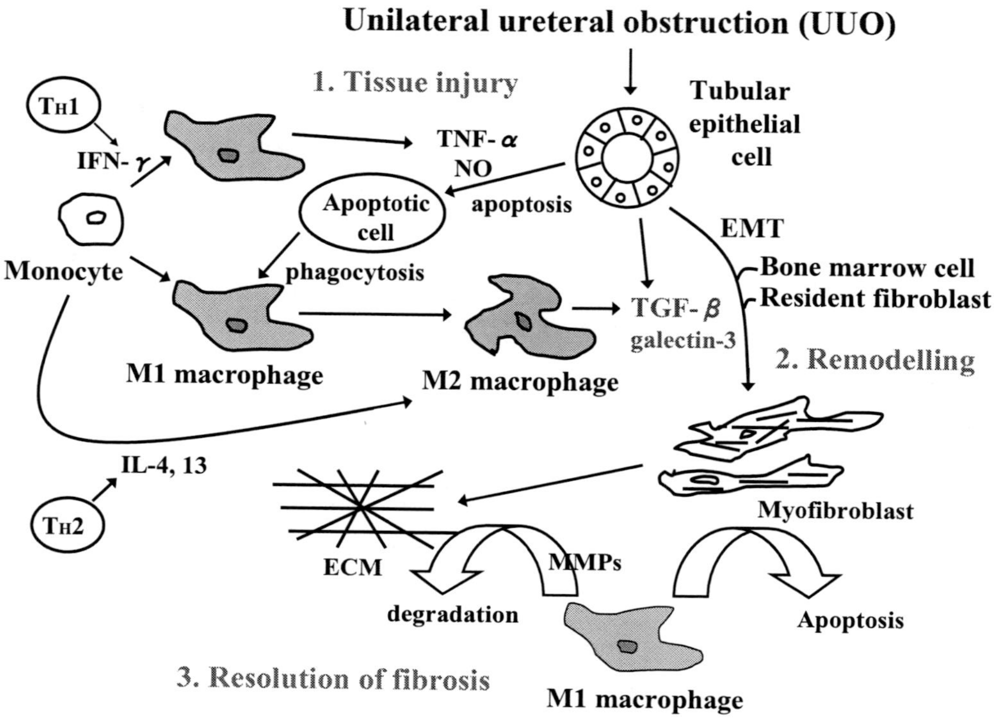

Figure 1. The regulation of fibrosis by macrophages in obstructed kidneys. Following UUO, recruited monocytes that differentiated into M1 macrophages produce pro-inflammatory mediators (TNF-α, NO) and induce tubular epithelial cell apoptosis and tissue injury. (1. Tissue injury) Then, the differentiation into M2 macrophages is induced and M2 macrophages generate anti-inflammatory cytokines such as TGF-β and galectin-3 that result in myofibroblast proliferation and ECM deposition. Tubular epithelial cells, bone marrow cells, and resident fibroblasts are the source of myofibroblasts. (2. Remodelling) ECM accumulation and matrix degradation products stimulate the differentiation into M1 macrophages, which produce MMPs that promote ECM degradation and induce apoptosis of myofibroblasts. These matrix degradation products and apoptotic debris are possibly removed by phagocytosis of M1 macrophages. (3. Resolution of fibrosis) UUO, unilateral ureteral obstruction; IFN-γ, interferon-γ; TNF-α, tumor necrosis factor-α; NO, nitric oxide; IL-4, interleukin-4; TGF-β, transforming growth factor-β; EMT, epithelial-mesenchymal transdifferentiation; ECM, extracellular matrix; MMPs, matrix metalloproteinases.

Conclusion

Although macrophages have classically been recognized as an active player in progressive renal scarring, several recent studies have suggested a renoprotective role of infiltrating macrophages that preserves renal architecture and limits progressive renal scarring in the late stage after UUO. These seemingly paradoxical findings may reflect the differential regulation of inflammation and fibrosis by two functionally distinct phenotypes of macrophages. Consideration on these phenotypes of macrophages is required in the analysis of the mechanism of renal fibrosis, and this may provide more detailed information regarding the disease status and prognostic evaluation in the biopsy specimens as the functional variation of these macrophages becomes more clearly defined. Furthermore, these macrophage phenotypes have important implications for therapeutic approaches to renal fibrosis. Macrophages are not committed to a single activation status during the inflammatory response that determine tissue injury or recovery, and novel therapeutic agents that specifically target either M1 or M2 macrophages may represent a more selective approach for renal fibrosis. The inhibition of M2 macrophages during progressive fibrosis would be predicted to decrease the fibrotic response. Recent studies discovered molecules that regulate alternative macrophage activation such as galectin-3 [31-33] which may provide new therapeutic targets. As an another therapeutic target, while IL-13 is associated with M2 polarity, the inhibition of IL-13 pathway by the IL-13 decoy receptor has been shown to decrease pulmonary fibrosis [34]. Since M1 macrophages may be anti-fibrotic, attempts to convert M2 macrophages to a M1 phenotype might be helpful. A caveat with this potential approach is that agents used to stimulate the M1 phenotype are pro-inflammatory and may induce tissue injury. Future work that further defines the molecular phenotypes of these macrophages will provide new macrophage-based therapies for renal fibrosis.

References

[1] Bascands JL, Schanstra JP: Obstructive nephropathy: Insights from genetically engineered animals. *Kidney Int* 2005; 68:925-937.

[2] Eddy AA: Interstitial macrophages as mediators of renal fibrosis. *Exp. Nephrol.* 1995; 3:76-79.

[3] Schreiner GF, Harris KPG, Purkerson ML, Klahr S: Immunological aspects of acute ureteral obstruction: Immune cell infiltrate in the kidney. *Kidney Int.* 1988; 34:487-493.

[4] Nishida M, Fujinaka H, Matsusaka T, Price J, Kon V, Fogo AB, Davidson JM, Linton MF, Fazio S, Homma T, Yoshida H, Ichikawa I: Absence of angiotensin II type 1 receptor in bone marrow-derived cells is detrimental in the evolution of renal fibrosis. *J. Clin. Invest* 2002; 110:1859-1868.

[5] Zhang G, Kim H, Cai X, Lopez-Guisa JM, Carmeliet P, Eddy AA: Urokinase receptor modulates cellular and angiogenic responses in obstructive nephropathy. *J. Am. Soc. Nephrol.* 2003; 14:1234-1253.

[6] Cochrane AL, Kett MM, Samuel CS, Campanale NV, Anderson WP, Hume DA, Little MH, Bertram JF, Ricardo SD: Renal structural and functional repair in a mouse model of reversal of ureteral obstruction. *J. Am. Soc. Nephrol.* 2005; 16:3623-3630.

[7] Nishida M, Okumura Y, Fujimoto S, Shiraishi I, Itoi T, Hamaoka K: Adoptive transfer of macrophages ameliorates renal fibrosis in mice. *Biochem. Biophys. Res. Commun.* 2005; 332:11-16.

[8] Pecly IM, Gonçalves RG, Rangel EP, Takiya CM, Taboada FS, Martinusso CA, Pavão MSG, Leite Jr M: Effects of low molecular weight heparin in obstructed kidneys: decrease of collagen, fibronectin and TGF-β, and increase of chondroitin/dermatan

sulfate proteoglycans and macrophage infiltration. *Nephrol. Dial Transplant.* 2006; 21:1212-1222.

[9] Nishida M, Okumura Y, Ozawa S, Shiraishi I, Itoi T, Hamaoka K: MMP-2 inhibition reduces renal macrophage infiltration with increased fibrosis in UUO. *Biochem. Biophys. Res. Commun* 2007; 354:133-139.

[10] Duffield JS: The inflammatory macrophage: a story of Jekyll and Hyde. *Clin. Sci.* 2003; 104:27-38.

[11] Mosser DM: The many faces of macrophage activation. *J. Leukoc. Biol.* 2003; 73:209-212.

[12] Wilson HM, Walbaum D, Rees AJ: Macrophages and the kidney. *Curr. Opin. Nephrol. Hypertens* 2004; 13:285-290.

[13] Lupher Jr ML, Gallatin WM: Regulation of fibrosis by the immune system. *Adv. Immunol.* 2006; 89:245-288.

[14] Ferenbach D, Kluth DC, Hughes J: Inflammatory cells in renal injury and repair. *Sem. Nephrol.* 2007; 27:250-259.

[15] Ricardo SD, Goor HV, Eddy AA: Macrophage diversity in renal injury and repair. *J. Clin. Invest.* 2008; 118:3522-3530.

[16] Wada T, Furuichi K, Sakai N, Iwata Y, Kitagawa K, Ishida Y, Kondo T, Hashimoto H, Ishiwata Y, Mukaida N, Tomosugi N, Matsushima K, Egashira K, Yokoyama H: Gene therapy via blockade of monocyte chemoattractant protein-1 for renal fibrosis. *J. Am. Soc. Nephrol* 2004; 15:940-948.

[17] Sung SA, Jo SK, Cho WY, Won NH, Kim HK: Reduction of renal fibrosis as a result of liposome encapsulated clodronate induced macrophage depletion after unilateral ureteral obstruction in rats. *Nephron. Exp. Nephrol.* 2007; 105:e1-9.

[18] Goerdt S, Orfanos CE: Other functions, other genes: Alternative activation of antigen-presenting cells. *Immunity* 1999; 10:137-142.

[19] Duffield JS, Ware CF, Ryffel B, Savill J: Suppression by apoptotic cells defines tumor necrosis factor-mediated induction of glomerular mesangial cell apoptosis by activated macrophages. *Am. J. Pathol.* 2001; 158:1397-1404.

[20] Kipari T, Hughes J: Macrophage-mediated renal cell death. *Kidney Int* 2002; 61:760-761.

[21] Lange-Sperandio B, Cachat F, Thornhill BA, Chevalier RL: Selectins mediate macrophage infiltration in obstructive nephropathy in newborn mice. 2002; 61:516-524.

[22] Fadok VA, Bratton DL, Konowal A, Freed PW, Westcott JY, Henson PM: Macrophages that have ingested apoptotic cells in vitro inhibit proinflammatory cytokine production through autocrine/paracrine mechanisms involving TGF-β, PGE2, and PAF. *J. Clin. Invest.* 1998; 101:890-898.

[23] Song E, Ouyang N, Horbelt M, Antus B, Wang M, Exton MS: Influence of alternatively and classically activated macrophages on fibrogenic activities of human fibroblasts. *Cell Immunol.* 2000; 204:19-28.

[24] Raes G, Noël W, Beschin A, Brys L, de Baetselier P, Hassanzadeh GH: FIZZ1 and Ym as tools to discriminate between differentially activated macrophages. *Dev. Immunol.* 2002; 9:151-159.

[25] Gibbs DF, Warner RL, Weiss SJ, Johnson KJ, Varani J: Characterization of matrix metalloproteinases produced by rat alveolar macrophages. *Am. J. Respir. Cell Mol.* 1999; 20:1136-1144.

[26] Mariani TJ, Sandefur S, Robby JD, Pierce RA: Collagenase-3 induction in rat lung fibroblasts requires the combined effects of tumor necrosis factor-α and 12-lipoxygenase metabolites: A model of macrophage-induced, fibroblast-driven extracellular matrix remodeling during inflammatory lung injury. *Mol. Biol. Cell* 1998; 9:1411-1424.

[27] Iredale JP, Benyon RC, Pickering J, McCullen M, Northrop M, Pawley S, Hovell C, Arthur MJ: Mechanism of spontaneous resolution of rat liver fibrosis. Hepatic stellate cell apoptosis and reduced hepatic expression of metalloproteinase inhibitors. *J. Clin. Invest* 1998; 102:538-549.

[28] Cheng S, Lovett DH: Gelatinase A (MMP-2) is necessary and sufficient for renal tubular cell epithelial-mesenchymal transformation. *Am. J. Pathol.* 2003; 162:1937-1949.

[29] Lutz J, Yao Y, Song E, Antus B, Hamar P, Liu S, Heemann U: Inhibition of matrix metalloproteinases during chronic allograft nephropathy in rats. *Transplantation* 2005; 79:655-661.

[30] Duffield JS, Forbes SJ, Constandinou CM, Clay S, Partolina M, Vuthoori S, Wu S, Lang R, Iredale JP: Selective depletion of macrophages reveals distinct, opposing roles during liver injury and repair. *J. Clin. Invest* 2005; 115:56-65.

[31] Henderson NC, Mackinnon AC, Farnworth SL, Poirier F, Russo FP, Iredale JP, Haslett C, Simpson K, Sethi T: Galectin-3 regulates myofibroblast activation and hepatic fibrosis. *Proc. Natl. Acad. Sci. USA* 2006; 103:5060-5065.

[32] Henderson NC, Mackinnon AC, Farnworth SL, Kipari T, Haslett C, Iredale JP, Liu FT, Hughes J, Sethi T: Galectin-3 expression and secretion links macrophages to the promotion of renal fibrosis. *Am. J. Pathol.* 2008; 172:288-298.

[33] Mackinnon AC, Farnworth SL, Hodkinson PS, Henderson NC, Atkinson KM, Leffler H, Nilsson UJ, Haslett C, Forbes SJ, Sethi T: Regulation of alternative macrophage activation by galectin-3. *J. Immunol.* 2008; 180:2650-2658.

[34] Fichtner-Feigl S, Strober W, Kawakami K, Puri RK, Kitani A: IL-13 signaling through the IL-13α_2 receptor is involved in induction of TGF-β1 production and fibrosis. *Nat. Med.* 2006; 12:99-106.

In: Nephrology – Dialysis - Transplantation
Editors: Endre Kruger and Kelemen Hahn
ISBN 978-1-60741-736-1
© 2009 Nova Science Publishers, Inc.

Chapter X

Whence Forth after the GWAS Wave for Diabetic Nephropathy?

Daniel P. K. Ng[*1]
Department of Epidemiology and Public Health,
National University of Singapore, Singapore

Abstract

Two decades have passed since the first reports were published proposing that risk for diabetic nephropathy may be genetically determined. Since then, efforts using the candidate gene approach and conventional genome linkage scans have met with limited success. The feasibility of performing genome wide association studies (GWAS) has been realized in recent years and results from these on diabetic nephropathy will soon be available.

These studies will undoubtedly throw light on the involvement of novel genes in the pathogenesis of this complication. Nevertheless, it is also expected on the basis of the collective GWAS experience so far that these genes will have limited effect sizes (ORs typically <1.4). Furthermore, these genes will account for a very small proportion of the genetic risk. Importantly, it is quite unlikely that they are responsible for the linkage signals that have been observed in specific chromosomal regions of the human genome. Sieving the wheat consisting of both major genes purportedly lying in the linkage regions as well as additional minor genes from the chaff will continue to be challenging.

Keywords: diabetic nephropathy, genome-wide association studies, haplotype, major susceptibility genes, single nucleotide polymorphism.

---

[*] Corresponding Author: Daniel P K Ng, PhD. Department of Epidemiology and Public Health, Yong Loo Lin School of Medicine, National University of Singapore, 16 Medical Drive MD3. SINGAPORE 117597. SINGAPORE. Tel: +65 6516 4967. Fax: +65 6779 1489. E-mail address: ephnpkd@nus.edu.sg

Abbreviations

ACE	angiotensin-I converting enzyme;
CRF	chronic renal failure;
ESRD	end stage renal disease;
GFR	glomerular filtration rate;
GWAS	genome-wide association studies;
LOD	logarithm of odds;
OR	odds ratio;
PROT	proteinuria;
SNP	single nucleotide polymorphism;
UAE	urinary albumin excretion

Built upon the foundations of the Human Genome Project and the International HapMap Project, and coupled with advances in large-scale genotyping technologies, research collaborations that have pooled together sizable patient DNA collections have led to the recent spate of genome-wide association studies (GWAS) [1, 2]. With little known of the new susceptibility genes identified, GWAS will undoubtedly leave an indelible footprint on the human genetics landscape, serving to remodel our understanding of a host of complex diseases. A prime example of such a substantive impact is in the case for type 2 diabetes where a number of novel genes for this disease have been identified and convincingly replicated, paving the way for a subsequent dissection of their function and cellular pathways [3-9].

Diabetic nephropathy is the most severe microvascular complication of diabetes and is the major contributor to cases of end stage renal disease (ESRD) in many developed countries. Familial clustering consistent with the involvement of genetic risk factors has been thoroughly demonstrated [10]. Collaborative efforts at GWAS have been forged, consolidating cases and controls with either type 1 or type 2 diabetes [11-14]. These new GWAS results are already forthcoming, with preliminary analyses implicating regions on 11p15 and 9q22 as potentially harbouring these novel susceptibility genes [15]. This current round of GWAS will therefore enhance the pioneering but nevertheless limited efforts in that have been previously reported in this field [16-18].

However, one may already anticipate certain limitations from these new findings by drawing on the general collective GWAS experience for various chronic diseases [1]. Firstly, the implicated risk alleles will have modest effect sizes with typical odds ratios (ORs) <1.4 [1]. Secondly, the risk alleles will be quite frequent in the population, commonly >0.20 [1, 19]. Put together, this implies that the risk alleles will have a low penetrance since many individuals will carry the risk alleles but yet among these, the vast majority will continue to remain disease-free. Thirdly, the genes identified will be expected to merely explain a limited proportion of the familial clustering observed for diabetic nephropathy.

Critically, it is likely that the current GWAS wave will fail at unmasking the major susceptibility genes for diabetic nephropathy. These major genes are thought to lie in specific human chromosomal regions that show genetic linkage to diabetic nephropathy or its related traits of albuminuria and renal function. Several of these regions have been independently replicated such as those on 2q, 3q, 7p, 7q, and 18q (Table 1).

Table 1. Chromosomal regions exhibiting genetic linkage to renal traits in diabetes

Region	Traits	Type of diabetes	Reference
1q	GFR	Type 2	[41]
2p	GFR	Type 2	[41, 42]
2q	PROT, ESRD, UAE, GFR,	Type 1, Type 2	[27, 43, 44, 45]
3p	GFR	Type 2	[42]
3q	PROT, ESRD	Type 1, Type 2	[28, 46, 47, 48]
5q	PROT, ESRD	Type 2	[32]
6q	GFR	Type 2	[27, 49]
7p	ESRD, GFR	Type 2	[27, 28, 49]
7q	PROT, ESRD, UAE, GFR	Type 2	[32, 41, 45, 47]
8q	GFR	Type 2	[41, 42, 49]
10p	PROT, ESRD	Type 2	[45, 50]
10q	GFR	Type 2	[27]
11p	GFR	Type 2	[41]
14q	PROT, ESRD	Type 2	[45]
15q	UAE, GFR	Type 2	[41, 45]
16q	GFR	Type 2	[49]
17p	GFR	Type 2	[49]
18p	GFR	Type 2	[27]
18q	PROT, ESRD, GFR	Type 2	[28, 41, 45, 51]
19q	PROT, ESRD	Type 1	[43]
20p	PROT	Type 1, Type 2	[43, 47]
22q	UAE	Type 2	[32]

ESRD, end stage renal disease; PROT, proteinuria; GFR, glomerular filtration rate; UAE, urinary albumin excretion.

The reason for this apparent failure of GWAS has remained elusive. Still unproven is one possibility that while the risk allele in these major susceptibility genes would presumably be associated with larger effect sizes (i.e. greater ORs), the risk alleles may potentially be much less frequent although still more common than the rare mutations that characterize monogenic disorders. Despite their commendable sample sizes, this reduced allele frequency may have inadvertently reduced the power of current GWAS studies and hindered investigators from ascribing formal statistical significance to these associations particularly after correction for multiple hypotheses testing. Performing meta-analyses of individual GWAS studies coupled with large-scale replication has been helpful in identifying additional minor genes of even smaller effect sizes (ORs < 1.2) but its utility for pinpointing the major susceptibility genes has not been realized [20]. Sieving the wheat consisting of both major and minor genes from the chaff will undoubtedly continue to be challenging.

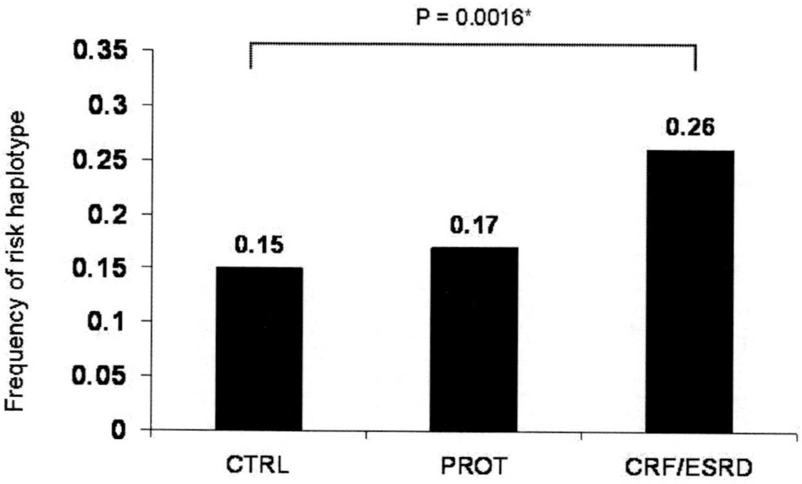

Figure 1. An IL-6 haplotype confers risk for ESRD but not proteinuria in type 2 diabetes [33]. CTRL, controls with normoalbuminuria; PROT, cases with proteinuria; CRF/ESRD, cases with CRF or ESRD due to diabetic nephropathy. *P < 0.05 after taking into account multiple haplotype testing.

Another noteworthy point is that the analyses of GWAS data are now primarily confined to the level of individual single nucleotide polymorphisms (SNPs). Correspondingly, there has been a lack of an unbiased genome-wide haplotype analysis. This deficiency is perhaps due to the computationally demanding nature of such a large scale haplotype analysis. Still, the results from some candidate gene studies of late have provided some grounds for encouragement to make progress on this front. For example, the well-known insertion/deletion polymorphism in the gene encoding for the angiotensin-I converting enzyme (ACE) is not strongly associated with diabetic nephropathy except upon undertaking a large meta-analysis [21, 22]. With a haplotype analysis using tagging SNPs, however, a robust association between ACE and diabetic nephropathy has been shown across independent studies comprising either type 1 or type 2 diabetic patients. This is despite sample sizes which are considered relatively modest by GWAS standards but adequate for candidate gene studies [23, 24]. Imputation of genotypes at un-typed SNPs by combining the knowledge of linkage disequilibrium patterns between SNPs (e.g., from the International HapMap project or resequencing data in a candidate region of interest) with actual genotype data at tagging SNPs collected on a phenotyped study sample, may supplement the current lack of haplotype analyses at the genome–wide level [25, 26].

A more recent report provides greater persuasion for hunting down potential major susceptibility genes in chromosomal regions linked to diabetic nephropathy. Two genome linkage scans had earlier revealed evidence for a gene locus on human chromosome 7p21 that was linked to ESRD and variation in glomerular filtration rate (GFR) [27, 28]. Ordered subset analysis showed significant evidence for linkage with ESRD (logarithm of odds, LOD = 3.6) in the 37% of African American families with longest duration of type 2 diabetes prior to onset of ESRD (28). In Caucasian families with type 2 diabetes [27], variation in GFR as estimated by serum cystatin C was also linked to this same locus (LOD = 4.0) with the peak of linkage co-localizing almost exactly with that reported among African Americans [28]. Inspection of the critical region underneath the peak of linkage revealed interleukin-6 (IL-6) as a prime positional candidate gene since chronic inflammation has emerged as a key pathway underlying the development of diabetic nephropathy [29-31].

Keeping in mind that these two genome scans had highlighted the linkage of 7p21 with renal function but not albuminuria [27, 28, 32], it is worth mentioning that an IL-6 haplotype has been exclusively associated with chronic renal failure (CRF)/ESRD but not proteinuria in a subsequent case-control study [33]. Besides the presence of an association which withstood the conservative Bonferroni correction, two other observations were pertinent. The estimated frequency of the risk haplotype was fairly high although less than that typically observed for SNPs identified through GWAS. Moreover, carriers of this risk haplotype had nearly twice the risk of ESRD compared to the other haplotypes combined [33].

In conclusion, when the current GWAS wave subsides, the challenge for the research community is clearly laid out if one subscribes to a prevailing view that major susceptibility genes may potentially exist. An even path towards achieving this goal however remains to be illuminated. More than a decade ago, it had been proposed that the positional candidate approach will become the predominant avenue for identifying such susceptibility genes in chromosomal regions linked to disease traits once the Human Genome Project has been realized [34]. Although largely left in the shadows due to the present interest in GWAS, this prediction may still materialize. Genomic convergence approaches that utilize additional sources of biological information such as catalogues of the urinary proteome as well as genes expressed in the glomerulus and its constituent cells may allow for a more judicious choice of positional candidate genes for investigation [35-40]. With a deeper mining of the ever expanding GWAS datasets both in terms of patient DNA collections and number of SNPs being probed, a more nuanced appreciation of what actually constitutes the clinical phenotype that is diabetic nephropathy could break the present deadlock and unveil the identities of these elusive major susceptibility genes.

Funding

Funding for D.P.K.N. is provided by the Singapore National Medical Research Council (NMRC/1018/2005).

Conflict of Interest

The author has no involvements that might raise the question of bias in the work reported or in the conclusions, implications or opinions stated. The results presented in this paper have not been published previously in whole or part, except in abstract format.

References

[1] Manolio T.A., Brooks L.D., Collins F.S. (2008). A HapMap harvest of insights into the genetics of common diseases. *J Clin Invest, 118,* 1590-1605.

[2] Prokopenko I., McCrathy M.I., Lindgren C.M. (2008). Type 2 diabetes: new genes, new understanding. *Trends Genet, 24,* 613-621.

[3] Diabetes Genetics Initiative of Broad Institute of Harvard and MIT, Lund University, and Novartis Institutes of BioMedical Research, Saxena R., et al. (2007). Genome-wide association analysis identifies loci for type 2 diabetes and triglyceride levels. *Science, 316*, 1331-1336.

[4] Scott L.J., Mohlke K.L., Bonnycastle L.L., et al. (2007). A genome-wide association study of type 2 diabetes in Finns detects multiple susceptibility variants. *Science*, *316,* 1341-1345.

[5] Zeggini E., Weedon M.N., Lindgren C.M., et al. (2007). Replication of genome-wide association signals in UK samples reveals risk loci for type 2 diabetes. *Science*, *316*, 1336-1341.

[6] Sladek R., Rocheleau G., Rung J., et al. (2007). A genome-wide association study identifies novel risk loci for type 2 diabetes. *Nature*, *445*, 881-885.

[7] Steinthorsdottir V., Thorleifsson G., Reynisdottir I., et al. (2007). A variant in CDKAL1 influences insulin response and risk of type 2 diabetes. *Nat Genet*, *39*, 770-775.

[8] Yasuda K., Miyake K., Horikawa Y., et al. (2007). Variants in KCNQ1 are associated with susceptibility to type 2 diabetes mellitus. *Nat Genet*, *40*, 1092–1097.

[9] Unoki H., Takahashi A., Kawaguchi T., et al. (2008). Single nucleotide polymorphisms in KCNQ1 are associated with susceptibility to type 2 diabetes in East Asian and Danish populations. *Nat Genet*, *40*, 1098–1102.

[10] Ng D.P.K., Krolewski A.S. (2005). Molecular genetic approaches for studying the etiology of diabetic nephropathy. *Cur Mol Med*, *5,* 509-525.

[11] The Family Investigation of Nephropathy and Diabetes Research Group. (2003). Genetic determinants of diabetic nephropathy: The family investigation of nephropathy and diabetes (FIND). *J Am Soc Nephrol*, *14 (7 Suppl 2)*, S202-204.

[12] Knowler W.C., Coresh J., Elston R.C., et al. (2005). The Family Investigation of Nephropathy and Diabetes (FIND): design and methods. *J Diabetes Complications*, *19*, 1-9.

[13] Mueller P.W., Rogus J.J., Cleary P.A., et al. (2006). Genetics of Kidneys in Diabetes (GoKinD) study: a genetics collection available for identifying genetic susceptibility factors for diabetic nephropathy in type 1 diabetes. *J Am Soc Nephrol*, *17*, 1782-1790.

[14] Unoki H., Kobayashi M., Araki S., et al. (2008). Identification of a new susceptibility gene to diabetic nephropathy in Japanese subjects with type 2 diabetes. *American Society of Nephrology 2008 Renal Week* (http://www.abstracts2view.com/asn/view.php?nu=ASN08L1_1610a) [Abstract]

[15] Pezzolesi M.G., Poznik G.D., Mychaleckyj J.C., Paterson A.D., Barati M.T., Klein J.B., Ng D.P.K., Placha G., Canani L.H., Bochenski J., Waggott D., Merchant M.L., Krolewski B., Mirea L., Wanic K., Katavetin P., Kure M., Wolkow P., Dunn J.S., Smiles A., Walker W.H., Boright A.P., Bull S.B., DCCT/EDIC Research Group, Doria A., Rogus J.J., Rich S.S., Warram J.H., Krolewski A.S. (2009). Genome-wide Association Scan for Diabetic Nephropathy Susceptibility Genes in Type 1 Diabetes Mellitus. *Diabetes,* 58, 1403-1410.

[16] Tanaka N., Babazono T., Saito S., et al. (2003). Association of solute carrier family 12 (sodium/chloride) member 3 with diabetic nephropathy, identified by genome-wide analyses of single nucleotide polymorphisms. *Diabetes*, *52*, 2848-2853.

[17] Shimazaki A., Kawamura Y., Kanazawa A., et al. (2005). Genetic variations in the gene encoding ELMO1 are associated with susceptibility to diabetic nephropathy. *Diabetes*, *54*, 1171-1178.

[18] Hanson R.L., Craig D.W., Millis M.P., et al. (2007). Identification of PVT1 as a candidate gene for end-stage renal disease in type 2 diabetes using a pooling-based genome-wide single nucleotide polymorphism association study. *Diabetes*, *56*, 975-983.

[19] Doria A., Patti M.E., Kahn C.R. (2008). The emerging genetic architecture of type 2 diabetes. *Cell Metab*, *8*, 186-200.

[20] Zeggini E., Scott L.J., Saxena R., et al. (2008). Meta-analysis of genome-wide association data and large-scale replication identifies additional susceptibility loci for type 2 diabetes. *Nat Genet*, *40*, 638-645.

[21] Ng D.P.K., Tai B.C., Koh D., et al. (2005). Angiotensin-I converting enzyme insertion/deletion polymorphism and diabetic nephropathy: A meta-analysis of studies reported during 1994-2004 and comprising 14,727 subjects. *Diabetologia, 48*, 1008-1016.

[22] Ng D.P.K., Tai B.C., Lim X.L. (2008). Is the presence of retinopathy of practical value in defining cases of diabetic nephropathy in genetic association studies? The experience with the angiotensin-I converting enzyme I/D polymorphism based on 53 studies comprising 17,791 subjects. *Diabetes, 57*, 2541-2546.

[23] Ng D.P.K., Placha G., Choo S., et al. (2006). A disease haplotype for advanced nephropathy in type 2 diabetes mellitus at the angiotensin-I converting enzyme gene locus. *Diabetes, 55*, 2660-2663.

[24] Hadjadj S., Tarnow L., Forsblom C., et al. (2007). Association between angiotensin-converting enzyme gene polymorphisms and diabetic nephropathy: case-control, haplotype, and family-based study in three European populations. *J Am Soc Nephrol*, *18*, 1284-1291.

[25] Servin B., Stephens M. (2007). Imputation-based analysis of association studies: candidate regions and quantitative traits. *PLoS Genet*, *3*, e114.

[26] Yu Z., Schaid D.J. (2007) Methods to impute missing genotypes for population data. *Hum Genet*, *122*, 495-504.

[27] Placha G., Poznik G.D., Dunn J., et al. (2006). A genome-wide linkage scan for genes controlling variation in renal function estimated by serum cystatin C levels in extended families with type 2 diabetes. *Diabetes*, *55*, 3358-3365.

[28] Bowden D.W., Colicigno C.J., Langefeld C.D., et al. (2004). A genome scan for diabetic nephropathy in African Americans. *Kidney Int*, *66*, 1517-1526.

[29] Shikano M., Sobajima H., Yoshikawa H., et al. (2000). Usefulness of a highly sensitive urinary and serum IL-6 assay in patients with diabetic nephropathy. *Nephron*, *85*, 81-85.

[30] Stehouwer C.D., Gall M.A., Twisk J.W., et al. (2002). Increased urinary albumin excretion, endothelial dysfunction, and chronic low-grade inflammation in type 2

diabetes: progressive, interrelated, and independently associated with risk of death. *Diabetes*, *51*, 1157-1165.

[31] Saraheimo M., Teppo A.M., Forsblom C., et al. (2003). Diabetic nephropathy is associated with low-grade inflammation in type 1 diabetic patients. *Diabetologia*, *46*, 1402-1407.

[32] Krolewski A.S., Poznik G.D., Placha G., et al. (2006). A genome-wide linkage scan for genes controlling variation in urinary albumin excretion in type 2 diabetes. *Kidney Int*, *69*, 129-136.

[33] Ng D.P.K., Nurbaya S., Ye S., Krolewski A.S. (2008). An IL-6 haplotype on human chromosome 7p21 confers risk for impaired renal function in type 2 diabetes. *Kidney Int*, *74*, 521-527.

[34] Collins F.S. (1995). Positional cloning moves from perditional to traditional. *Nat Genet,* 9, 347-350.

[35] He L., Sun Y., Takemoto M., et al. (2008). The glomerular transcriptome and a predicted protein-protein interaction network. *J Am Soc Nephrol, 19*, 260-268.

[36] Takemoto M., He L., Norlin J., et al. (2006). Large-scale identification of genes implicated in kidney glomerulus development and function. *EMBO J, 25*, 1160-1174.

[37] Adachi J., Kumar C., Zhang Y., et al. (2006). The human urinary proteome contains more than 1500 proteins including a large proportion of membrane proteins. *Genome Biol*, *7*, R80.

[38] He L., Sun Y., Patrakka J., et al. (2007). Glomerulus-specific mRNA transcripts and proteins identified through kidney expressed sequence tag database analysis. *Kidney Int, 71,* 889-900.

[39] Patrakka J., Xiao Z., Nukui M., et al. (2007). Expression and subcellular distribution of novel glomerulus-associated proteins dendrin, ehd3, sh2d4a, plekhh2, and 2310066E14Rik. *J Am. Soc Nephrol, 18,* 689-697.

[40] Nair V., Iyengar S.K., Sedor J.R., et al. (2008). Integration of gene expression with gene association studies in diabetic nephropathy. *American Society of Nephrology 2008 Renal Week* (http://www.abstracts2view.com/asn/view.php?nu=ASN08L1_1508a) [Abstract].

[41] Schelling J.R., Abboud H.E., Nicholas S.B., et al. (2008). Genome-wide scan for estimated glomerular filtration rate in multi-ethnic diabetic populations: The Family Investigation of Nephropathy and Diabetes (FIND). *Diabetes, 57,* 235-243.

[42] Freedman B.I., Bowden D.W., Rich S.S., et al. (2008). Genome-wide linkage scans for renal function and albuminuria in type 2 diabetes mellitus: the Diabetes Heart Study. *Diabetic Med, 25,* 268-276.

[43] Rogus J.J., Poznik G.D., Pezzolesi M.G., et al. (2008). High-density single nucleotide polymorphism genome-wide linkage scan for susceptibility genes for diabetic nephropathy in type 1 diabetes: discordant sibpair approach. *Diabetes, 57,* 2519-2526.

[44] Puppala S., Arya R., Thameem F., et al. (2007). Genotype by diabetes interaction effects on the detection of linkage of glomerular filtration rate to a region on chromosome 2q in Mexican Americans. *Diabetes, 56,* 2818-2828.

[45] Iyengar S.K., Abboud H.E., Goddard K.A.B., et al. (2007). Genome-wide scans for diabetic nephropathy and albuminuria in multiethnic populations: The Family Investigation of Nephropathy and Diabetes (FIND). *Diabetes, 56,* 1577-1585.

[46] Moczulski D.K., Rogus J.J., Antonellis A., et al. (1998). Major susceptibility locus for nephropathy in type 1 diabetes on chromosome 3q: results of novel discordant sib-pair analysis. *Diabetes, 47,* 1164-1169.

[47] Imperatore G., Hanson R.L., Pettitt D.J., et al. (1998) Sib-pair linkage analysis for susceptibility genes for microvascular complications among Pima Indians with type 2 diabetes. *Diabetes, 47,* 821-830.

[48] Osterholm A.M., He B., Pitkaniemi J., et al. (2007). Genome-wide scan for type 1 diabetic nephropathy in the Finnish population reveals suggestive linkage to a single locus on chromosome 3q. *Kidney Int, 71,* 140-145.

[49] Chen G., Adeyemo A.A., Zhou J., et al. (2007). A genome-wide search for linkage to renal function phenotypes in West Africans with type 2 diabetes. *Am J Kidney Dis, 49,* 394-400.

[50] Iyengar A., Fox K.A., Schachere M., et al. (2003). Linkage analysis of candidate loci for end-stage renal disease due to diabetic nephropathy. *J Am Soc Nephrol, 14,* S195-S201.

[51] Vardarli I., Baier L.J., Hanson R.L., et al. (2002). Gene for susceptibility to diabetic nephropathy in type 2 diabetes maps to 18q22.3-23. *Kidney Int 62,* 2176-2183.

Index

A

B

C

D

E

F

G

H

I

M

N

O

P

Q

R

S

T

U

V

W

X

Y